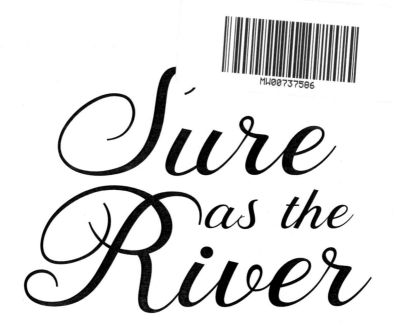

Sure as the River

Wandering Back to Saskatchewan

C. Sloan

CHARLOTTE EVELYN SLOAN

ISBN   978-1-7775187-6-9 (Hardcover)
ISBN   978-1-7775187-4-5 (Paperback)
ISBN   978-1-7775187-5-2 (EPUB)
ISBN   987-1-7775187-7-6 (Kindle)

Editing & Proofreading Services, Lantern Hill Communications

Published by Marmie's Corner

First Edition: February 2021

Dedicated to my girls,
Angie and Carrie

Blessed are the pure in heart, for they shall see God.

CONTENTS

THE FIRST DAY

"**C**ome in with me, Ralph, please." We could read the sign by the door of the red brick building – HOME FOR UNWED MOTHERS.

"I told you before, I can't. They have their rules."

I stared at him in disbelief. I saw his fingers gripping the steering wheel as if his life depended on it. He waited, looking perturbed. "Hop out quick and take your bag. Get inside as soon as you can."

I felt like a rebel child pleading with my eyes, with my heart, with my soul. "You're better than this Ralph, way better, and you know it. You could at least have the decency to come in with me. You're dropping me off like a dog."

He looked away from me, staring straight ahead at the street. He was eager to hit the gas and get on out of there.

"I promise I'll come in a week or two. Don't sign anything. I meant what we talked about, Liz. Just go up the steps and get in there. People are watching." Now he was the one pleading.

My last words to him were, "I see more and more of your dad in you." It wasn't a compliment.

I took a deep breath. It was hard to appear dignified as my belly was sticking out so far, I couldn't see my shoes. I had no words. I hurried up the wooden steps towards the black and white sign, pressed the doorbell, and as instructed, opened the door and disappeared inside.

I knew the car was already speeding away. "Thank you, Ralph Parker," I muttered. "Do you know what you've done?"

An ominous black dress was coming towards me, and the noise of heels clicked on the tiled floor. Determined to start on the right foot, I extended my hand. "Hi. I'm Liz. Liz Parker."

She ignored my greeting and my proffered handshake. She looked me up and down with obvious disdain, her eyes focusing on my midsection. She directed me to follow her, and we hurriedly retraced her steps down a long, dark hallway. I held onto my small suitcase, and with an overwhelming sense of trepidation, I entered her office.

A sign on her desk gave her the distinction of "Director". After two or three minutes in her office, I got the message loud and clear - I was scum, and she was the queen of this dubious castle. Alarm bells were clanging somewhere in my head as she outlined the rules of her well-run establishment. Ridiculous! Unbelievable! Her black hair was pulled back so tightly, it had to be constricting her brain. First and foremost, she warned me not to utter my last name to anyone, ever. I should instead use only the initial of my last name.

I quickly spoke up. "My name is Parker and I am not ashamed of it."

She answered with a smirk, "Of course you're not ashamed of your name! Why would you be? But face it, your family is ashamed of you."

An instant frown burrowed into my forehead. I thought of my dead mother, whom I could not remember. She was hardly ashamed of me!

The director added, "Keeping your name to yourself is to protect them from your shame."

Them? Who was she talking about? Not my mother. Not my dad, in his tight coffin since 1940, when Ralph took over the farm. No, he didn't care two hoots all my life, and he didn't need to be protected from me now, even if he had still been breathing. That left Ralph.

"Are you referring to my brother, Ralph?"

"Precisely."

"And you think he's ashamed of me? Really? How would you know that?"

Her beady eyes roved over my body once again, remaining on my protruding belly. I met her gaze. She gave the impression that my appearance repulsed her. I knew I did not have movie star looks. I was not Rita Hayworth or Ginger Rogers, but there was nothing about me to warrant that look. I had often been told that I was attractive. My brown eyes matched my naturally curly hair and I had a wide, winning smile. I wore a crisp, blue dress I had sewn myself, from a pattern my aunt and I had created. It had a drawstring channel at the waist that allowed room for expansion. I had made two more that were similar, but in different colors.

The director referred again to Ralph's impression of me. "Common sense tells me a lot. We see your kind in here day in, day out."

She shoved a form across the desk and nodded sharply, not bothering to ask me to fill it out. At the top in the first blank, I wrote the date, October 17, 1943.

Age: 20

Occupation: Seamstress and companion to an elderly woman.

How many months pregnant? 7

Marital status: Single

Are you here of your own will? I circled the word, "Yes".

What are your intentions regarding your baby? I printed in large block letters so there would be no mistake: TAKING MY BABY HOME WITH ME. I then signed the spot marked "Signature" and pushed the paper back towards her.

She snatched it up and at a glance saw what she was looking for. Obviously, the information she wanted was the "intention".

"We'll see about that! You must know a bastard child has no hope in society. We advise all the women who come through here to relinquish their baby for adoption to give it a chance for a respectable and successful life."

Her speech sounded like a script she had memorized and took delight in reciting one more time. By now I was fired up. Ralph had dumped me in a prison and this warden was planning to take my baby. I stood to my full height. My aunt, with whom I had lived for the past 12 years, had insisted on good posture despite my being taller than most girls. I was much taller than the director and she looked shriveled in every sense, sitting behind her desk, twirling her fountain pen.

I could see the checklist on her desk. "Did you bring any money with you?"

"I have $20."

"You'll turn it over to us, and it will be returned the day you leave."

I did not make a move to hand it over. She stared at my white clutch purse and touched a small dome bell near her ink bottle. A younger woman entered and said, "I work in accounts. We both sign this, confirming the amount and the date."

I was in a daze as I handed her two tens, and she and I both signed before she quickly left. My mind was whirling in wild circles. Before we drove up to the address, I had been off and on in my dilemma, whether to take my money in with me or leave it in Ralph's care. On a last-minute impulse, I folded the envelope and tucked it into his jacket pocket.

"Don't cheat me out of it, Ralph. It represents 12 years' wages!"

As I gave up my twenty dollars, I thanked my lucky stars that at this moment Ralph had the keeping of my money. I trusted him more than these crooks. I was sure I'd never see those two purple tens again!

I was not yet aware of all the rules, but the truth was dawning.

"Depending on your attitude, contact with friends and family is limited." I had planned to keep in touch with Aunt Flo and with Ralph and his wife, Irene.

Disbelief washed over me. This place, these women, were bent on rendering me powerless without a cent in my pocket, with no contact to the outside, and without even my last name. In less than a half-hour, they had stripped me of my identity!

I felt the need to defend myself. "I've been taught to respect myself and others." She sniffed, a very significant sniff and we both knew the interpretation. I continued, "I refuse to stay where I am not respected."

She looked up at me, challenging. "So, you're a tough one, are you Liz? Many a woman comes here and has the decency to be grateful for a place to hide her shame, give birth, and go away with a lesson learned."

I said nothing.

She continued, "Some are fighters. You may as well know right now, the rules here are rigid and unbending. Don't cross me. It won't go well for you.

"Put her in Room 18," she ordered a sour-faced young woman who stood in the doorway. There was no please or thank you in this place. No common decency. I followed the warden's assistant back through the dim hallway. As soon as we entered the room, I looked at the staff woman and mustered a smile. "My name is Liz." I purposely left off my last name. When she didn't respond, I said, "Where I come from, introducing yourself is considered polite."

All she said was, "The less you share with the women in here, the better. The bathroom is down the hall - we passed it on our way. When you go in there, make it snappy. There's always someone waiting."

I was done talking. She added, "Put your things in the dresser and your suitcase under the bed."

I was relieved when she turned away from me and scuttled down the dark corridor. Since she apparently didn't have a name, I gave her one - Miss Ewe. Like a sheep, she didn't have a mind of her own, but followed the orders of the despicable "powers that be". I had no desire to settle in, so I left my suitcase unopened. I sat on the bed for a few minutes, then kicked off my shoes and stretched out on the covers to rest my back.

It had been a long drive to this god-forsaken place, starting very early in the morning. Saying goodbye to Aunt Flo had been more difficult than I could have imagined. This morning a dark curtain of uncertainty had hung over both of us.

Her home had been my home since I was eight years old, and we had come to think of it as "our home" and the two of us as "family". With both our futures up in the air, this was the long goodbye. Ralph was tapping the palm of his hand on the doorknob, urging our departure. My gaze swept the old, familiar room. Memories, mostly fond memories, rose in my throat. Ignoring Ralph's impatience, I knelt by my aunt's chair.

"Bless me, Aunt Flo. I'm shaking in my boots."

With uncharacteristic tears, she whispered, "I do bless you, Child. You're the strongest person I've ever known. Go in peace!"

It was the strangest parting. This woman had been my rock, my shelter, my teacher, and my support since I was a child. I came to her from under a doctor's care. I had been injured at the hand of my father, and Ralph was the one to come home and find me beaten, bloody, and with a broken arm. After medical treatment, Ralph arranged for our Aunt Flo, Dad's oldest sister, to take me in.

She did not have children, and so my boisterous laughter and childish behavior must have been a shock to her system. I was a fun-loving kid, in spite of my abusive childhood. I had a broad toothy grin, as when my permanent teeth came in, they were too large. What can you do? I don't remember worrying about that.

My aunt was prim and proper. She was small in stature, yet commanded respect from the whole town. Twice a year her friend Mabel came to the house to give her a perm. The pink box with grey stripes had the word "Toni" on it, and the contents, once mixed together, stunk up the entire house. She endured the rows of little paper-covered curlers soaked in the Toni solution for the prescribed time and by the end of it all, she had tight little grey curls all over her head. She didn't wash her hair for well over a week so the perm would "take", and it did seem to last the full six months. She sewed her clothes, using choice fabric and the perfect trim of lace or piping. No matter the occasion, her appearance was always more than presentable. She insisted on me being neat and tidy, but she did allow me to wear slacks because she knew I'd be climbing fences, running with the Rogers kids, and doing our outside chores.

Over the years, I learned so much from her. She taught me to be polite and decent. She also passed on her "trade" to me - all the know-how and the intricacies of being a seamstress. We derived an income from our sewing, and she was wise in the way of finances. We managed better than most. Her war widow's pension saw us through what people called the Dirty Thirties. She was of the mind (and passed that on to me) that if a job is worth doing, it is worth doing well. Aunt Flo saw to it that I became an excellent housekeeper, an admirable cook, and a woman with confidence. We had made a go of it through thick and thin, best times and hard times. She wasn't healthy, but I was, and I was already used to working hard when I moved in. I had done my best, and so had she.

This morning it all came to an end. My last glimpse of her is printed in my mind - head bowed, showing her tight, grey curls, shoulders back, eyes closed, tears slipping down her cheeks. It wasn't supposed to end this way for us. My aunt forced out of her home to be taken in by family, as she had done for me 12 years before. And here I was, embarking on a path I never dreamed I would be on, alone and pregnant. The Home for Unwed Mothers was the last place I expected to be.

In a half-hour, my three roommates entered Room 18. I sat up, feeling better than I had when I lay down. None of them spoke to me. One last try.

"Hi, I'm Liz."

The women each said their first name. I have never put up with uncomfortable silence in my life, and I said to no one in particular, but to all of them at once, "What kind of a place is this? I've only been here an hour and it feels like a house of horrors."

One girl volunteered, "We're not supposed to talk to one another."

"I've been to a lot of places in my lifetime, but this is the closest place to hell that I've ever experienced." My roommates looked horrified, as if I could be shot by a firing squad for saying that. The same girl who said we weren't to talk, mouthed the words, "It's safer after lights out." Then she said aloud, "Right now we go for supper."

I crammed my swollen feet into my shoes and joined the others as we silently filed out the door to wherever the dining room was. Sure enough, Miss Ewe appeared from nowhere. I had no doubt she had been spying on us, to see if they would talk to me.

Late at night, the girl who said we were not to talk to each other, padded over to my bed. She put her head on the edge of my pillow so I could hear her whisper, "I'm pleased to meet you, Liz. I'm Grace No-Name, and we'll find a way to be friends."

Relieved, I smiled at her in the dim, shadowy light. "Thank you, Grace. I can't believe this place."

"I know. Don't fight them, Liz. You can't win. The director probably failed to tell you that our mail is censored, and we are not free to come and go."

"I'm not surprised. It's a hell hole if I ever saw one."

As my tired body relaxed and sleep became inevitable, a song came to my mind. I had been a music lover for as long as I could remember. I knew all the current songs and who sang them. If my situation hadn't been so tragic, I would have been amused at just how appropriate the words were when Tommy Dorsey's popular song came floating into my mind, "I'll Never Smile Again". It was a grim thought to go to sleep on.

And so ended my first unspeakable day at the Home for Unwed Mothers. My last day there came sooner than expected, and it was just as shocking, and much more terrifying.

THE LAST DAY

On November 29, I woke up after a rough night. I was sweating profusely and I ached everywhere. Still three weeks to go till my due date, and I wondered how much longer I could hold on. I had long since been "rotated" to another room. In fact, this was my third. Grace and I were not allowed to be roommates or to sit together at meals, as the staff deemed that we were getting too friendly. The goal was to keep us alone and lonely.

At the moment, I wasn't thinking about Grace or anything else except how sick I felt. The girls had already left our room to be on time for breakfast. I slowly dressed, shuffled down the long hallway, and almost lost my balance, landing heavily on a bench near the front door. Whether it was a coincidence or providence, at the very same time someone from the outside rang the doorbell and banged loudly on the door. The warden clicked her way towards the commotion, her eyes shooting daggers. As she reached for the door handle, she spied me on the bench.

"Get!" She spat out the word as if I were a stray dog. I didn't move. I'm not sure I could have.

The banging continued, and she yanked open the door, fire breathing through her nostrils, ready to do battle. There were no appointments this early in the morning.

Unbelievably, in walked my brother Ralph, all six foot, three inches of him. He took in the scene in seconds - I, almost passed out on the bench, and the warden huffing and blowing, trying to block his way. Ralph looked stunned. His head swiveled from me to her, her to me, and back again. "What in blazes have you done to my sister?"

The warden was quick to answer. "She's pregnant! She did it to herself." I have laughed since at her ridiculous statement. I suppose there are still people who think unwed mothers manage to get that way on their own. At that moment, no one was laughing. I tried to say something, but my voice was not there. I had been feeling rough for a couple of weeks, but nothing as bad as this.

Ralph yelled at the warden. "What have you done? Look at her swollen neck, and her eyes bugging out of her head. Get a doctor in here right now!"

The lady in black didn't hesitate, but hurriedly began dialing the wall phone near my bench. I am not sure if she was afraid of Ralph, or if she had taken a careful look at me because of Ralph's command, and knew something was badly amiss.

Ralph knelt on the floor beside me. "Oh Sis, what did they do to you?" I was suddenly back on the ground by our house on the farm, eight years old and unable to move. Ralph had come to my rescue that day, and ended up placing me in Aunt Flo's care. Now this morning, once again it was my big brother Ralph who showed up when I needed him most.

I closed my eyes and drifted away. The last I heard was Ralph shouting, "Forget the doctor! Get an ambulance!"

That was my final day in the warden's prison. I woke up days later to a new chapter of my life, and I never looked back.

WHERE AM I?

I opened my eyes to see a high, white ceiling above me. Where am I, and why am I here? I may have asked those two questions out loud, as immediately a male face popped into my vision, his eyes close to mine.

"Good morning Liz! I'm Dr. Sanders."

Slowly, memory took shape. I touched my throat, and felt thick padded bandages. My hand went to my midsection and I knew I was no longer pregnant. I closed my eyes. I didn't want to see this Dr. Sanders. I didn't want to be here. I wished I was dead.

The doctor was happy to see me awake. He eagerly pulled a chair up to the rails on my bed and explained. "You've been sedated for days, Liz. Welcome back."

I didn't want to be back.

"You've been a very sick lady, and you're lucky to be alive."

Lucky? I doubt it.

"You've had emergency surgery. You're in the hospital and we're going to get you well again."

If he expected me to chat, I had no energy for it. I lay there staring at the high ceiling.

"A lot has happened in the past few days, and I'll explain it all to you as best I can. What do you want to know first?"

"Only one question, Dr. Sanders. Did they get my baby?"

He took my hand and said very softly, "Your baby is safe in the care of your relatives. She is small because she came early, but she's healthy."

That was all I needed to know. Ralph. My only relative, so he must be the one. My brother had rescued me twice in my life, and now apparently, he had also saved my child. He and Irene talked to me before I went to the Home for Unwed Mothers, and said they would be happy to adopt the baby. I told them there was not a chance in the world for that. Ralph knew my fierce nature, and I assured him I had money to help me get started as an unmarried mother, and I could do it on my own. I was a hard worker and nothing could stop me. Now, apparently, it all turned out just as they wanted. I lay there helpless to digest the information.

I guess I did have another question for the doctor. "What's wrong with me?"

"You have a condition called Graves' disease."

I had to say it. "It is appropriately named."

Dr. Sanders was proving to be a compassionate man with a ready smile. "It was first described a hundred years ago by an Irish doctor, Robert Graves. It commonly affects women under 40, and it's not cured, but rather treated. It has to do with an overactive thyroid gland, which can have very serious repercussions, as it has with you."

"And what did I do to bring this on?"

"Nothing at all, Liz. It can happen to anyone. It is sometimes traced to genetics, but in the medical papers I have recently read, they suggest it occurs more often when the patient is under emotional or physical stress. Interestingly enough, pregnancy can also trigger it."

With that information, my unfortunate pregnancy took on an added sinister aspect. The emotional stress I could and would forever blame on the director of the Home for Unwed Mothers, but the pregnancy? Responsibility for that lay at my own feet.

"Do you remember leaving the Home the day you were so sick?"

I answered, "No, I only remember my brother yelling for an ambulance."

I felt Dr. Sanders' sympathy. "I'll pick up the story from there, as much as I understand it. You were in real danger, as your thyroid gland had become so enlarged it was cutting off your breathing, and emergency surgery saved your life. The director of the home is being investigated, as she is responsible for the medical care of the women who stay there, and they are to have regular checkups by a physician. A doctor should have caught the problem long before it got to that stage.

There is still a report to come from that hospital regarding the birth of your baby. Apparently, though, she is well. That is great news, as often the mother's Graves' disease has serious effects on the baby. It does say in your file you experienced agitation, confusion, psychological disturbance, and mania. That's why you were transferred here."

"And where exactly is 'here'?"

"You're in a psychiatric ward in the provincial hospital."

"You mean the... mental?" I could hardly say the word.

"Some people call it that."

"Was I acting crazy?"

"It's a result of the hormones being way out of balance. As I told you, we're going to help you get well."

This news was a blow like nothing else. It struck somewhere in my soul, nothing like the abuse I had received from my father. Nothing like the cruelty of the director. This was shattering. I closed my eyes.

"The baby?"

"You were deemed incompetent because of the mania. Your next of kin legally took the child."

"And he sent me here?"

"He did. This is the best place for you right now, Liz. Mainly because I and a couple of doctors are up on Graves' and hyperthyroidism. We've had marked success with treatment. It will take a few months to get you healthy again, and other hospitals won't keep you that long. This is a suitable placement. Things will get better and better. Graves' often settles down after the initial episode. Then we keep a close watch on symptoms using medication and treatments."

Dr. Sanders was not so very many years older than I, but he patted my hand in the same way a grandfather would comfort a child. He left the room after telling me he would be back the next day. I was heartsick and every other kind of sick. I had landed in the mental!

Later in the day, I shuffled to the nearby bathroom with a nurse supporting me on either side. Unfortunately, there was a small mirror over the sink. When I stood there to wash my hands, I caught a glimpse of a pitiful excuse for a human being, looking back at me with mournful, bulging eyes. I forgot the nurses were there beside me. I gripped the sink with both hands, and I spoke each word very slowly, to the freak in the mirror, "*You* are not Liz Parker!"

Dr. Sanders came, again and again, trying to coax me into a conversation. One morning he asked, "Who are you, Liz? I'm trying to figure you out."

So far, I had avoided his probing questions, but on this day a little of my former spunk surfaced.

"You want to know? Well, I'm not *this*!" I pointed to my face. "Not at all this thin-haired, bug-eyed old woman! I'm a 20-year-old girl with naturally curly brown hair and normal eyes. I'm a hard worker, and I miss my job slinging out pastries and pouring coffee in the Air Training School café."

Dr. Sanders said, "We're getting you sorted out Liz, little by little. Surgery didn't take all of your thyroid gland because you do need some of that hormone. That partial surgery is called in medical terms a "subtotal thyroidectomy". The positive news is surgery is a sure way to get your system back on track and is the fastest way to restore hormone levels."

I asked him about my voice. "I used to be a good singer. I think I may have lost that, too."

"I don't think so. Your voice is stronger and better now than it was right after surgery, so I doubt any serious damage was done. It will take time. Singing will come back. You'll have to practice, but I guess you first need to feel like it."

That was true. There was no song in my heart.

"You are making exceptional progress, Liz. Your nurses say the sweating is decreasing, the hand tremors are less pronounced, and you're gaining a little weight. And even though there is so much for you to be anxious and irritable about, you are calmer than you were."

I asked the unspeakable question, and I dreaded his answer. "What about my eyes, Dr. Sanders?"

Quick to spout a wealth of knowledge about Graves' disease, he replied, "About half of Graves' patients develop moderate to severe "exophthalmos", which is a medical term for protrusion of the eyeballs. It increases moderately after surgery. What it is, is swelling and inflammation of eye tissue."

In all of his fancy explanations, I did not hear one word about my eyes getting back-to-normal. I felt his compassion as he asked, "Do your eyes hurt you, Liz?"

I answered quickly, "Only when I look in the mirror."

Dr. Sanders specialized in treating patients at the hospital with hyperthyroidism. As the months passed, he continued to encourage me. I pondered his comment, "In years to come, we will do a much better job of treating patients with thyroid hormone issues. Even now in the '40s, some are treated with radioactive oral medication. Considering how severe your onset was, I feel that you have responded well to the partial surgery and to the medication we are giving you. It's called thiouracil, and it has nicely replaced your restlessness and emotional issues with calm composure. If you find that you just don't cry, that's why."

I asked how long I would have to stay in the hospital. He took a long time to respond, and then said he thought if I felt strong enough, I could move to another part of the hospital. The area I was in was designated for medical patients who needed constant nurses' and doctors' supervision. He felt I was ready to go to a job each day, along with the hundreds of residents of the hospital. He said it would do me good to be busy and productive.

"So, you're kicking me out?"

"Oh no, not at all, Liz. I will see you from time to time, and we will still carefully monitor your medication and symptoms. We want to keep on top of your thyroid levels. We'll move you over to the Women's Ward tomorrow."

THE WOMEN'S WARD

I didn't mind the prospect of trying another place. Perhaps the doctor was right, and meaningful work would help my outlook on life and the future. I couldn't sleep a wink all night. I was trying to process the past. I didn't even know for sure on what date my baby had been born. I wondered about my Aunt Flo. For the very last time, I sifted through the details of the months that led up to our separation and the awful twist my life had taken.

I met Ray at Christmas, 1942. The war affected our everyday lives, and we were all taken by surprise when the Air Training Schools quickly sprang up across the country. The one nearest to us opened in the fall of '41, and hundreds of pilots and their instructors landed in town. Suddenly, there was fun and festivities, dances and dates, something for all of us. If we didn't know how to dance, we learned, and finally, after the hard times of the Depression and the rations of the war, we could lighten up. Of course, the war was still raging overseas, and we were still under heavy ration restrictions, but the air force had come to us. With it came privileges we hadn't seen in a long while. There were jobs galore, and Carl Rogers offered rides to whoever needed a lift into Stillwater, as our town was a few miles out. I started doing volunteer work at the coffee shop, and soon I had a part-time paying job, serving coffee and snacks to handsome men in uniform.

Ray Hutton arrived in December, and we hit it off right from the start. He called me Smiley, no doubt because of my toothy grin, but I didn't care. Carl's sister and I loved to dance, and so did Ray. We laughed a lot. At one time I said I thought we were getting too serious. He put his arm around me and said, "No way Liz! You're my girl, and nothing will change that."

The winter months went by. News of the war was front and center in all of our minds, keeping track of which local boys had joined up. It was common for their mothers to share blue airmail letters right then and there in the post office with anyone who was interested. We sent packages overseas containing cigarettes, chocolate bars, soap, socks, combs, and gum. We knew some parcels wouldn't arrive, but we did our best to cheer on our home town boys. Monthly Red Cross blood clinics were held in the basement of the United Church. The community suffered as one.

It was a different way of living, and not only for the boys overseas. Even here at home on the Prairies, there was a feeling of tension in the air that couldn't be described. The future was uncertain, and many of my friends embraced a devil-may-care attitude. Anything could happen, anywhere, anytime.

The schedule at the flying school was rigorous. New guys were rolling in on the trains, and business was booming in the town. Ray usually picked me up on a Saturday night at seven. He didn't have a vehicle, but he was a persuasive guy, wheeling and dealing, trading cigarettes and who knows what, to borrow a car when he wanted one. One Saturday night, I waited till almost eight o'clock, puzzled as to where he was, and a little worried, as he always drove too fast.

The phone rang. Ray's voice was different, sort of strained, and excited at the same time. "Hello, Love. I'll get straight to the point. I'm not coming tonight."

"Aw Ray…"

"The air force has come between us, Liz. We always knew it would. Those big wigs we saw all week holding meetings and interviews were making their selections. A group of us have just had a briefing. We're on our way out on the morning train."

I was speechless. He was right. We both knew he would be going sometime. That was the whole point of coming to the training center in the first place, to get further instruction and flying hours in before being sent to the front.

"So, I won't see you?"

"I can't help it, Love. Duty calls!"

I could tell he wasn't at all sad to be leaving me. This was his dream, and he was ecstatic. I didn't mean a pin to him.

"We had some plans, Ray."

"We did, but this isn't the right time to be making promises, Liz. I might not make it back, and that's a fact. And you might get tired of waiting. It's wartime, after all."

I had planned to tell him that I was pregnant when he picked me up. I thought we'd talk about getting married. I tried to sort my thoughts. Should I tell him? I decided not.

"Have a swell time tonight, Ray. I can hear the party warming up!"

He stammered a little and said, "It's just the guys here, Liz. You know how they are." I could hear girls laughing, and lots of shouting and fooling around. I hung up the phone. What a stinking excuse for a man, and what a stinking fool I had been. I should have known. It's wartime after all!

I wondered why I had left it so long to tell Ray about the baby. Maybe something in my subconscious knew he was not the type to stay. "Good Time Raymond", that's what they called him at the flying school.

THE BEGINNING
OF THE END

I was about five months pregnant, and my aunt was no fool. After supper on a Saturday night, two weeks after the final call from Ray, I poured mint tea into her favorite china cup. I had a mug I liked for myself. It wasn't fancy, but I could wrap my fingers around its warmth. Mint was growing everywhere in our yard. The old Depression years of drought were gone and our garden was lush and green.

Not in my usual hurry to clear the table, we stayed where we were, both tired. The evening light came through the west window and showed the lines on her face that had appeared in recent weeks. I asked if she had been having heart spells lately, and she answered, "Some."

"Aunt Flo, we need to talk."

"Yes, we do. You go first."

I hated the shadow that crossed her face when I told her. I had often overheard her praising me to the neighbors and to her friends affirming our relationship, and how I was a better seamstress than she was, and twice as fast. She loved me not only for my skills and for our teamwork. We were a family, a World War I widow, and a 20-year-old foolish girl, but we were family all the same.

"If you haven't guessed already, Aunt Flo, I'm pregnant."

She hadn't guessed. I saw the shock and pain darken her eyes, but only for a moment. I couldn't bear that look.

"I've disgraced you, after all these years of you training me to be a decent human being."

She gave me a look of pure love. It was a weak and understanding smile that I did not deserve.

"You've not disgraced me, girl. That has nothing to do with me. You've made things hard for yourself."

"Don't I know it!"

The tick-tock of the clock on the wall by the window marked the passing minutes.

"Now it's your turn, Aunt Flo. I bet you can't top that!"

"Well, it's all changed now, what I was going to say. It's changed in these last few seconds. I had decided it was time to give in to the pressure from my sister and move out to BC to live with her. It looked to me like you were needing your freedom."

"What I'm needing is your help to get through this."

She nodded. "Tongues will wag. This town and any other town will have no mercy. We'll fend them off together, and we'll find a way."

Summer ended, and the cold prairie winds of October rattled the dry cornstalks in our garden. I was feeling better than I had at the beginning of my pregnancy. I had been so dog-tired during the first three months, but with the urgency of getting the yard and garden produce tucked away for winter, and taking care of fall housecleaning inside, I mustered the energy I needed. Worry for my aunt hung heavy on my mind. I often heard her coughing in the night, and I slowly and silently opened her door to see if she needed me.

It was also in October that we received a letter in the mail from the village office. This was unexpected, as our mayor was a long-time friend of my aunt, and lived three houses down on our street.

I seldom saw Aunt Flo angry through the years, though I had seen her firm and no-nonsense side come out every once in a while. I had more often seen her kind and generous nature, such as when she boarded the neighbors' cow when they had no feed in the '30s. But the day she read that letter, I saw her ripping mad. It fell from her hands onto the table as if it were a hot coal. I picked it up and read it aloud. As if she needed that!

"Dear Florence Melbourne,

This letter is to give notice of the termination of your lease of property Lot 1, Block 4, Village of Cala, as of November 30, 1943.

This property rental was granted to you in 1917, due to your status as a WWI widow, having been married to Sgt. Jack Melbourne, now deceased. Due to the critical housing shortage at this time, your current tenancy has been re-allocated to a returning wounded veteran.

Sincerely,
Frank Hamilton, Mayor, Village of Cala"

"It's because of me, isn't it?"

She nodded. "No doubt."

My pregnancy was obvious, and I had made no pretense of hiding it. I did all the shopping and errands that needed doing, as Aunt Flo didn't have any energy to spare. Well, they 'had' us. As far as finding a solution, the timing was not on our side. That night she had a spell with her heart, gasping for air as I phoned for the old doctor who lived in the center of town. In the morning, we put in a call to the relatives in BC. Her sister was delighted. I could hear her across the room, "We'll take care of one another, Flo. This is my dream come true."

It certainly wasn't my dream! I needed to move within days, but I had no clue where to go. I was feeling poorly, my hands were shaky, and I often had sweats. I didn't know that was part of being pregnant.

My aunt called me into her room very late that night. She had two things to say.

"Excellent news, Liz. I've contacted your brother. He's making arrangements for you at the Home for Unwed Mothers, where you can wait till the baby is born. By then, he and Irene will have something set up for you."

I didn't have much choice. I had made a little money earlier in the summer working at the coffee shop, but when Raymond left town, I quit going near the place. There was talk of it soon closing down.

My aunt continued. "One more thing, Girl. I have money for you. You've worked like a slave all through these years, and I have some wages for you."

I protested, although there was probably never a time in my life that I would need it as desperately.

"I can't take it."

"Oh yes, you can. Nobody's getting this except you. And don't worry about me. My sister married a banker and she's loaded. I'll be fine."

She pointed to a fat envelope on the nightstand. "Take it, Liz. It's yours. You'll need it for the little one. I wish we could do this together, but you heard Doc say it. My heart is giving out."

Things happened swiftly after that. My aunt gave most of her belongings to her friends, and one by one, they happily came and drove away with what had constituted the necessities and comforts of our home. I packed her personal items in one suitcase, and mine in another. I didn't have much to take - the bulging envelope of money, clothes, and a few personal effects. Ralph came for me by the end of the week. The rest was history.

As my sleepless night in the Medical Ward ended, I detected a rosy glow in the small window across from my bed. A new day was dawning. I had no idea what the Women's Ward held for me. I promised myself I would not re-live again my goodbye with Ray or with my aunt. It was all in the past.

Before noon, I was moved to an area of the hospital I had not known existed. I was to share a room with three women. I could tell the room was already crowded with three, but they had moved in a bed and a small night table for me. I had no belongings of my own. I did not know it then, but I was about to get my education about this massive brick complex they called the Asylum for the Insane.

WORK THERAPY

W hen I first entered the hospital, I was placed in a small medical ward. That space was a mere drop in the bucket, compared to the vast configuration of added wings and attached buildings. When I passed a large, framed photograph displayed on the wall, I was amazed to see how huge the place was.

All my life, I had known about the "Mental", at least that it existed. I had seen it from the highway, as its tall chimney was visible for miles. It was not unusual to see a work crew cutting and gathering hay in the ditches as we passed by. I didn't give it a thought back then. I just knew where they were from. A man from our town had gone to the hospital for treatments and came home doing fine. A woman was admitted there, and we never saw her again. Now, unbelievably, I was here myself as a patient, and I was still reeling with the reality of it.

The three roommates were not talkative, and neither was I. Ironically, there was no restriction on our conversation here, yet we had nothing to say. Back at the Home for Unwed Mothers, we were aching to have someone's ear, to cry on a shoulder, to ask questions, and to find comfort, but we weren't allowed. Life had turned upside-down. I was on an unfamiliar planet with no hope of escape, and even if I could get out, where would I go?

I was given a canvas dress that was unattractive and stiff, along with underclothes, socks, and shoes. The shoes were too small. I wondered where my clothes were, especially those pretty new dresses I had sewn for myself with the expanding waistlines. Someone somewhere had my shoes, my purse, and my stockings.

A staff person wearing a light-colored uniform escorted me to the laundry. It was a huge area with machines and steam and no end of women milling around, dressed exactly as I was, in grey shapeless dresses.

"We start most women off in the laundry," my supervisor explained, "just to see if you know how to work." She set me to the task of removing wet laundry into large tubs on wheels and that's what I did all day long, except during a lunch break. I was on the chain gang, as much in prison as I had been under the director's nose.

A small bag containing soap, comb, toothbrush, towel, and washcloth, was packaged and on my bed when I returned to my room after supper. I found a nightgown folded under my pillow.

The room was tight. There were two beds on either side of the room, the ends touching. All my life I had a compulsion to be friendly and to set people at ease. My usual greeting was, "Hi, I'm Liz." I had no interest in greeting them. Exhaustion settled over me, and I could hardly force my blistered feet to take me to the bathroom, where I washed my face and brushed my teeth.

As we undressed for bed, I said nothing to the ladies, and they said nothing to me. When the lights went out, one of them, the old one on my side of the room, started mumbling to herself. The volume increased steadily until she was yelling. "Henry! Henry! Get your ass in here!" We ignored her, and as suddenly as she had begun the racket, she flopped back on her pillow and began to snore.

As the days passed, I noticed the women working in the laundry were as slow as molasses in January. I had always been a quick worker, and my aunt had praised me for it. She used to say, "Liz, you get more done in a day than two men and a boy." I realized the monotonous labor in the hot, steamy laundry would never be finished. It would be the same drudgery one day after another. I slowed my pace, and methodically put in only the effort that was expected of me.

After a week, a nurse came to our room and told me I would be taken to see Dr. Sanders after breakfast. I felt a flicker of hope, I'm not sure why, except that he was the one person who knew my name. He asked me how my work assignment was progressing, and I told him it would be a lot easier if my feet weren't blistered and bleeding. He asked me to slip off my shoes, and I bent down in my chair to pry them off my feet.

I was sure I saw a look of disgust flash across his face, but he smiled and said, "Well, this is ridiculous! We can do better than that." He nodded to the nurse sitting on a chair beside me, taking notes. Away she went with the offending shoes, leaving me with my feet curled back under my chair.

Dr. Sanders removed the bandage from my throat and said, "Oh yes, the surgeon did a fine job." He grabbed a hand mirror from a table that had various instruments on it, and held it so I could see the bright red scar that was healing well. I could tell it was healed enough to go uncovered. Another unsightly detail exposed.

The doctor continued in his extra chipper tone. "We'll check your thyroid levels, Liz. You're looking well, and I think the test will show we are making progress with the medication you're taking. By the way, have you made any friends over there in the Women's Ward?"

He acted like the world was all sunshine and roses, but I saw through it and his enthusiasm seemed forced.

I answered honestly, "No, am I supposed to?"

He was doing his best. "Well, a friend is a good thing to have."

I agreed with him. "I know, I've had many."

The nurse returned with a basin of warm water and gauze bandages. She knelt on the floor to bathe my feet. I felt a rush of emotion as she washed first one foot and then the other, and patted them dry with a small towel. She applied medicated salve and the gauze, and carefully put a white ankle sock on each foot.

As she stood to her feet, I caught her eye. "Thank you. Thank you so much."

She pointed to the larger shoes she had placed on the floor for me to try on. I did, and they felt fine. Just right, even with the socks.

I could tell Dr. Sanders was ready to wrap up this little visit, so I quickly spoke up. "I have a question. How long will the Graves' treatment take?"

He understood I was asking when I could get out, but he answered exactly what I asked. "It usually takes one to two years to get the thyroid hormones leveled out. We'll monitor carefully for a few months, and then make a plan for long term treatment."

I had lost track of time. No one mentioned what day it was, and I was struggling to remember what month. It is confusing when you lose that handle. We didn't work on Sundays, and that was a small anchor for me.

As an afterthought, Dr. Sanders asked, "How's the work going for you?"

"I am an excellent seamstress, Dr. Sanders. If there is ever an opening in the sewing room, I would appreciate a promotion."

Someone was waiting in the doorway to escort me back to the Women's Ward. I thought I saw a meaningful look pass between her and the doctor. I was right, as when we got back to my ward, instead of turning right to the laundry, she turned left. She opened the door to an enormous room with rows of sewing machines, bolts of grey canvas fabric, irons, a pressing machine, and shelves filled with sewing notions. Sunlight poured in through the tall windows.

I was led to a desk near the door and was presented to the woman in charge. "Marj, this is Liz. She is an excellent seamstress and has requested to be part of your team."

I was impressed that my escort took my word for it and recommended me as "excellent". I had lost confidence in almost every area of my life. Of one thing I was certain - I was well able to handle whatever tasks Marj had for me. The sewing machine was calling my name, and I felt a glimmer of interest.

Marj was plump, with freckles on her arms and cheeks, and she had a friendly face. Her hair had once been some shade of orange or red. She set me to work right away, but appeared to be rushed with her workload, and wasted no time in idle chit-chat. The hum of the treadle sewing machine brought comfort to me, and my feet were thanking me for the shoes that fit.

Bit by bit, I learned about the hospital. It was a world within the real world, a well-oiled, self-sufficient machine. The whistle blew at mealtimes and for shift change. Hundreds of patients under a medical prescription of "heavy work therapy" worked long hours, and in so doing, provided food for all those living under the roof, including the staff. The patients had been skilled farmers, home-makers, and tradesmen before being admitted. Under their expertise, the gardens, orchards, and greenhouses yielded healthy fruit and vegetable produce, vital to sustain the population. Expert animal husbandry resulted in abundant provision of pork, beef, chicken, eggs, and milk. The laundry where I had worked each day served the entire hospital with washed sheets and towels and clean clothing for the patients. There was a shoe repair shop, Marj's gargantuan sewing area, which was comprised of several rooms, as well as a barbershop, and a beauty parlor. Whatever service was required, it was provided right there on the grounds. The place even generated its own water and electricity.

I wondered who the Mastermind was. Someone had to be at the top, efficiently organizing staff rosters, and these hundreds of people, while also treating them for their mental health. I escaped those treatments because of the Graves' disease. Dr. Sanders knew what was wrong with me, and my thyroid levels were controlled by medication. There was no need to put me through anything else.

Most of the patients were subjected to different types of hydrotherapy, electrotherapy, and of course, the "heavy work therapy" in which I also participated. Imagine calling it "therapy"! To me, it was free labor to keep the place running. I went so far in my suspicions, as to imagine they may keep some skilled patients there for the greater good, rather than discharging them back to their homes.

I had a lot of time to think as I worked long hours in the sewing room. Memories sifted through my mind. I hardly recognized myself. The girl I once was had disappeared, and like the one I called Miss Ewe back at the Home for Unwed Mothers, I followed the others. They didn't talk, I didn't talk. They didn't laugh, I didn't laugh. I systematically went through the workday with my regrets and my dreams locked inside. My Aunt Flo had taught me to do my best work, no matter the circumstances.

Marj often complimented me on my sewing. I wondered if she could be that friend the doctor had wished me to find. As time passed, I realized I was simply part of her job, and she no doubt had a real life and real friends elsewhere.

Dr. Sanders had taken time off from the hospital to study with some young medical researchers. He said they would be sharing exciting information on his favorite subject of Graves' disease. It didn't matter to me that he was gone. I felt attached to him when I first came because he treated me as a friend. He was caring and compassionate, but as time went on, I was well aware that he was the doctor, and I was the patient. At the end of the day, he put on his coat and went home. I had no home to go to, and returned through two sets of locked doors to the Women's Ward.

I was offered work in the mattress shop, where blankets and hair mattresses were made for the entire hospital. I turned it down. After taking a brief tour, I could see it involved heavy physical work, and it was mostly all men who were working there. I preferred to do what I did best under Marj's watchful eye.

Days, weeks, months… my July 18th birthday came and went. I saw a different doctor, who checked my thyroid levels. Graves' disease had taken its treacherous toll on me. I no longer looked like myself. It was a struggle to keep my sails up, to leave the past where it belonged, and to scrounge some hope for my future. Physically, I was feeling better. My hair had thickened up and got curly again. Overall, I was feeling quite well, but the loneliness was killing me.

THE BIG BOSS

One day I made a comment to my supervisor on the way to our noon meal, and the result was better than I could have hoped. All I said was, "I wish I could be outside more." I was allowed to go for group walks in the evenings when the weather was favorable, but I had always been an outdoors person, and the long hours inside were stifling.

Marj replied, "I don't see why you can't. There is always greenhouse and garden work to be done. I'm sure you're due for a change."

From that time on, after breakfast each day, I was taken through the series of locked doors to the great outdoors, and was set to work in the fresh air. To my surprise, the three women in my room were also taken there. Until then, I had no idea what they did all day or where they went. They were more talkative out there, energized perhaps by gardening, as they probably had done at their own homes in their previous lives.

While working in the greenhouse, I met a young woman by the name of Lily. She was a chatterbox if I ever heard one, and she was obsessed with information about the hospital. She asked if I knew what year it opened. I did not. So, we went from there.

"Well, it was in 1913, and it filled up really fast, too." Her next question, "Do you know why they make us work so hard in here?"

I noticed that she, in particular, wasn't working "so hard". She had been flitting from person to person all morning, quizzing them on various topics, mainly the hospital. When I thought back to my days at the laundry, I identified with the term "working so hard". I had seen the farmworkers, slowly making their way back to the building after a long day in the sun. I had observed exhausted patients falling asleep before they finished the evening meal.

Lily had the answer concerning the work. "It's because the Big Boss calls it heavy work therapy. It's to make us so tired that we sleep at night and don't think much about our problems. I listen a lot to the nurses, and they're always saying what the Big Boss wants next. He says no one can say the word "asylum" ever again. You can only say "hospital".

I remembered, when I asked where I was, Dr. Sanders said I was a patient in the provincial hospital. He disapproved of me calling it the Mental.

"The Big Boss likes giving us the treatments." I kept pulling weeds from the rows of carrots that were in a raised garden bed and put no strain on my back.

Lily was still wound up. "Have you ever had the water?"

"What water?"

"Well, you know, the water treatments. Hydro. Just your head is sticking out and they pour water on you for a long time. Some people like it."

I shrugged my shoulders.

"Then there are the bad ones, the electro ones, the shocks, but the Big Boss likes them, too. He thinks they fix people's brains."

I wondered where this walking encyclopedia got her information. The details were a little sketchy, but oh, it gave me a lift to have someone to talk to. I didn't find an opportunity to say much, but I realized how I had missed interacting. This girl Lily, in my past, would have been annoying, but today she was gold. She looked me over from head to toe, as if doing a medical exam.

"If you don't get the treatments, why are you here?"

I didn't mind her questions, though I was sure she would hurry off to tell someone else all about it. "I have to take medication for a condition I have."

"Oh, does it have anything to do with your eyes? They're sticking right out!"

"Yes, it does.

"Oh, that's nice."

I wondered what was nice about it. Lily came a little closer and pulled a few weeds and some carrots by accident along with them.

"Do you like being here?" she asked.

"No, not much."

"I like it here. I like the flowers and I like snooping around the wards at night."

I was horrified - and slightly amused. "You do?"

"Yes, I sure do. I see lots of interesting things you wouldn't believe."

"Lily, are you sure it's safe to prowl around this place at night?"

"Well, of course, I can only go in the Women's Ward 'cause we're locked up.

"I'd like to go to the morgue. Did you know there's a morgue? It's in the down-down-down basement. I think it's haunted."

I was pretty sure she was trying to shock me, so I answered calmly, "I don't believe in places being haunted. I think there are scary places and sad places, but not haunted."

"Oh, you'll find out at the full moon."

"Will I?"

"Yes, and there are cemeteries here, too, out in the dark."

"I've heard that."

"Good for you, you heard right!"

Suddenly, Lily was gone, and I could see her scurrying along the path to where the older ladies were picking peas into big metal buckets. Fresh peas would probably be on the menu for supper, at least in some of the dining rooms.

Lily was short, with straight, black hair and dark eyes. I could easily imagine her sneaking around at night, in places she had no business going. I could tell she was mischievous, and I believed her when she said she liked being at the hospital. I couldn't figure out her age, perhaps thirty.

She showed up again before the workday was done. This time, she was wearing a green garden hat that was too big, and I could barely see her eyes. I had a sneaking suspicion someone was missing their hat, but it wasn't my problem. She stared at me for a while, and then asked, "Did you do a lot of work today?"

I told her I had enjoyed the work. "I hope they let me come again tomorrow."

She said quickly, "Oh, they will. You just ask them. The Big Boss thinks you're a good garden woman."

After supper, I spoke to the ladies in our room. I mentioned I had seen them out in the garden. Not one of them answered. The one who had called for "Henry" the first night in the room was quieter now most nights.

We went to bed early. It took me hours to get to sleep, and I often thought of life as it was before, when I was a kid. I thought of Carl and my aunt, and the whole Rogers family. I blocked out Ray and the Air Training Plan. I blocked out thoughts of the director and Miss Ewe, and I blocked out thoughts of my brother, Ralph. The little joke I amused myself with was that I blocked them out, so I could stay sane while living in an insane asylum.

I wondered if I would be going back to the sewing room. But thankfully, the following morning after breakfast, I was in the group our supervisor led outside. It was another beautiful, sunny day, and I felt better than I had in months. Weeding flowerbeds was my assigned task. I took my time, and soaked up the heat on my back.

I wasn't surprised when Lily showed up again. She admired the flowers and picked some, then left them on the edge of the lawn.

"There are different wards for different people around here, you know. Of course, there's the Women's Ward (it's really big), and there's the senile ward." She was counting them off on her fingers. "And the mentally defective, and the TB wards, and the basement wards. They're the worst."

I moved on to the next flowerbed, where some women were transplanting red geraniums. Lily said, "I feel sorry for the old women who can't feed themselves. Sometimes I go help the nurses feed them supper. You should come, too."

I agreed to do so, if she would come and find me when it was time. Sure enough, after we ate, Lily appeared with a nurse, and we found our way to a room where several elderly women lay in their beds, with a waiting tray on each nightstand.

It was a pleasure to offer my services. I chatted with the lady, as she ate ever so slowly. I told her about the flowers and my work outside. Partway through, a nurse from the bedside near me, said, "You should have been a nurse."

I answered, "You're right. I should have been a lot of things."

Lily and I were taken back to the Women's Ward. Of course, we were escorted wherever we went, because of the locked doors. The one who said, "You should have been a nurse," was our escort. I felt guilty for my bitter remark. I cleared my throat and spoke to her as we walked.

"I owe you an apology. You gave me a compliment, and I was rude. It was nice of you to say it."

I could tell she was surprised. She smiled and said, "It's okay, I understand." A big load lifted off my shoulders.

I thanked Lily for suggesting we go feed the ladies.

"I heard you singing, as you served that restless lady by the window."

"I know. It calms her down when I sing."

I remembered Dr. Sanders telling me I should practice singing to get my voice back after surgery.

"Next time, Lily, I'll sing with you and we'll liven up mealtime for them."

Lily was quiet for a moment and then said, "When they shut down garden work in the fall, let's ask if we can do nurse work."

This girl was smart. Many would call her simple. I would call her compassionate and clever.

Suddenly, she was back to information about the hospital. "Everybody loves the stone chapel. Emile made it. Did you see it?"

I nodded. "But only on the outside."

"Do you like it here?" she asked.

I smiled at her. "As I told you yesterday, not so much."

"Well, I like it here. The red flowers are my favorite, and I like poking around in the dark. I think I might go searching tonight to see what I can see."

"Goodnight, Lily." I doubted she would go anywhere, except to her own room.

When summer turned to fall, our supervised outdoor walks were still allowed and encouraged, but the gardens and greenhouses were put to bed for the winter. It happened, just as Lily had suggested, that our request to work with the elderly ladies was granted. The nurses were eager for our help, and so we used our energy and our compassion to make life better for those who were bedridden. Serving them made life better for us. Aunt Flo had told me something I would never forget. She said when word came from the army that her husband had died in the war, she was numb initially, and couldn't see a way to go forward.

"I learned that when you are empty, you dig deep and you will find something, not for yourself, but something to give someone else."

My interaction with the old patients was working wonders in me. I was talking again, which made me feel more like "me". I sometimes laughed, just like I used to. Lily said my laugh reminded her of a horse out in the stables at the hospital. I hoped it wasn't that bad, but I didn't care. Having the ability to laugh again proved my broken heart was mending.

I met a kind and gentle lady by the name of Illa when I arrived at the hospital and worked in the laundry. She worked slowly and methodically. Her hair was pulled back in a bun, which accentuated her square jaw. She was quick to greet the patients and staff as we arrived for work each day.

My heart went out to her one morning, when she asked one of the supervisors when she might be allowed to go home again for a visit. Illa's eyes were filled with longing and hope as she posed the question. I stopped to eavesdrop, curious if they might grant her wish. The staff woman with pursed lips seemed to be annoyed with the question.

"Not much chance of that! Your constant whining about going home is exactly why it won't happen." Illa's face crumpled with disappointment. Like a child denied going to a birthday party, she turned slowly back to her task folding towels. I had heard her talking at the table during lunchtime. She spoke a lot about her home, the farm, and her parents. There was one brother she referred to as "our Bob." She also told whoever was interested, about a surgery she'd had. "Do you want to *thee* my *thcar*?"

I was surprised then, to meet up with Illa once again when Lily and I volunteered to feed supper to those patients who could no longer feed themselves. She looked weary after a day of work, but she was on the job, feeding Mrs. Dodds! They were a compatible match. Illa did everything slowly, and Mrs. Dodds required an extremely long time to finish her meal.

Lily and I sometimes sang together to make mealtime pleasant for all, and we soon noticed Illa humming along. She was a bit of a monotone, but after our rendition of "You Are My Sunshine", Illa volunteered to sing by herself. We encouraged her, and so like a little child performing, she stood up straight beside Mrs. Dodd's bed and began her solo. Her voice was thick, with a bit of a lisp, but we understood each word:

Jesus loves me this I know,
For the Bible tells me so.
Little ones to him belong,
They are weak but he is strong.

Mrs. Dodds, who seldom made a sound, joined in.

Yes, Jesus loves me,
Yes, Jesus loves me,
Yes, Jesus loves me,
The Bible tells me so.

I realized once again that my inner soul was healing. I was able to see and feel beauty at that moment. These two ladies, bereft of earthly charm, would have been shunned had they been out in society, but here they were in this safe place, singing with the angels!

I continued to assist the nurses as required. I was often called back to Marj's department to teach sewing procedures, or to help catch up on urgent projects. I liked the variety, and I realized I was moving with the rhythm of hospital life. Never in a million years did I dream I would be living this surreal existence, month after month.

I remembered Mrs. Ross telling another staff person that every report on Illa included the same line: "This patient longs for home." I assumed hundreds of files contained the same theme. I longed for home, too, but where was it? I no longer had a home, and even if they discharged me from the hospital, I had no place to go.

I was completely shut off from my previous existence. Anyone seeing me today would never know I was once a normal, well-liked young girl working with my aunt to put food on the table, and offering cheerful help to anyone who needed it. Instead, they would see me as a mental patient with bug eyes. Sometimes I saw myself the same way.

THOUGHTS OF
THE FUTURE

Near the end of the year, Dr. Sanders arranged a checkup for me. He had just returned from his research trip and was eager to share what he had learned about Graves' disease. I had very little interest in his discoveries, as I was confident that I was getting better and was hopefully "over it". As I entered the office, a nurse offered me a chair, and we waited for the doctor to come in.

He greeted me with a big grin and exclaimed, "Liz, you're looking terrific! I've read all the reports in your file, and I'm thrilled the medication has worked so well."

He handed over a deck of cards. They may have been from France, as they featured a picture of the Eiffel Tower on the back of each.

"I brought you a little present."

I had played crib and other card games with the Rogers kids back in our school days. I thanked him for his thoughtfulness. A game of solitaire now and then might be a welcome diversion. I then ventured to ask if he could clear up the time issue for me, as I was confused regarding the past months. He thumbed through my file.

"Well, Liz, you've been here for almost a year. You came in December, the end of 1943. The first three months, you were in the medical ward, and then the Women's Ward. You were in Laundry for a week in March, then on to the Sewing Department. And, it looks like you've spent the summer, from June onward outside in the gardens. That's excellent! You're looking so healthy! That just proves getting outside is so important."

He kept turning pages in my fairly thick file. "And the latest report says you are now assisting the nurses!"

I nodded and smiled. It was the best job yet, and I enjoyed it.

Dr. Sanders smiled, too. "I'm not the least surprised, Liz. Even back at the beginning, when you were very ill, I could tell you were a compassionate and kind lady."

I stood to signal the end of our meeting. The doctor had people to see and places to go.

"So, Dr. Sanders, can you just tell me the truth. Is this a life sentence for me?"

He turned his head sharply and asked me to sit down. "No Liz, you're not here forever. I have big hopes and dreams for my patients. It's not going to happen overnight, but change is inevitable. If I were to ask you right now what your deepest wish is for your future, what would you say?"

I had not expressed my thoughts on the matter to anyone, even though I thought about it every day. My answer was rather tentative. "I'd like a normal life…out there. I'd have a home of my own, friends, and a job I like."

Even as I said the words, they sounded hollow, expressing a ridiculous and unrealistic goal. I heard my own sarcastic laugh.

Dr. Sanders replied earnestly. "That's what I want for you, too, Liz, and I'm sure it will happen one day. We can't push patients out of here without a plan, but some hospital officials are already talking about how it can be done."

I listened intently, as he continued to share the possibilities. "Some patients come in here for treatments, and when they are well, are released to their families. That works well for them, because they already have supports. For others, like you, we need a plan. It may start with a small number of patients, who are ready and able to leave, but they will need their confidence restored. Our patients are part of a big, isolated community here, and will need some time to be reacquainted with the world out there. There is a suggestion that in the early stages, staff members, or perhaps interested community members, will get paid to take into their homes "out-patients" who come back to the hospital for social events, volunteer work, and health checkups. In that way, our patients can still be supported by the security of the hospital, but will also find their place in the community again."

A myriad of thoughts raced through my mind. Everyone I had known out there had no doubt moved on, while I had been stuck in this place, standing still. Dr. Sanders' look was so intense, reminding me of his efforts when I was first admitted, to cheer me up and make me want to live again. He took a deep breath.

"Do you want to hold on for that?" he asked.

I didn't have an answer but I did pose a question. "Dr. Sanders, where is my fine brother in all of this? Do you know?"

He looked at the floor, as if guilty. "It's my fault you haven't heard from him, Liz. I advised him that stress is a significant trigger for Graves' disease. I know you have issues with his wife, and of course, they have your child. I felt the risk was too great, until we have proven your stability."

"Was he willing to come?"

"Yes, of course, he was."

As I played a game of solitaire that evening, I had a lot to consider. If I bought into the doctor's hope for the future, the waiting might destroy me. I had already discovered that the wheels at the hospital turn very slowly.

My thyroid test results consistently came up as satisfactory. According to Dr. Sanders, I had passed an entire year in the hospital. This comment triggered various thoughts. My baby would have celebrated her first birthday. My aunt was probably in glory. The war continued, as far as I could tell from listening in on conversations with the staff. As the New Year approached, I had no thread of hope that I would ever return to the "real world".

LIVING, LEARNING, AND REMEMBERING

Years passed, and I was still there. A shroud of helplessness wrapped itself around me. One of Aunt Flo's well-used lines was, "There's always a way, you just have to find it." On this one, even my aunt's sure-fire wisdom fell short. If only I could turn back the clock! I wished to be a kid again, when life was easy and simple, playing hide-and-go-seek and sitting around a bonfire, fending off mosquitoes. Most of the kids in town played ball on summer Saturday afternoons, and often parents showed up with a picnic lunch for us after the game. Back then, I had dreams of becoming an independent adult. Instead, I was now tied up as tightly as our cow, Bally, at milking time.

I spent a lot of my time remembering the details of my childhood. When I moved into my aunt's house in the town of Cala, I was eight years old. The house had a clean and peculiar smell, which I later found to be the wax she used on the shining linoleum floors. The house was neat as a pin, with everything in its place. Cushions were perfectly arranged on the couch, and ornaments on side tables, the likes of which I had never seen before. At bedtime, she led me to the guest room, as she called it, and turned back the covers for me. The quilts were exquisite, handmade, and colorful. I had never been a guest anywhere before, and I felt shy. The dresser in the corner had a large square mirror, but I could see only my face in it, as it was tilted to reflect a taller person. The bed was high, with two feather ticks on the mattress.

When Aunt Flo came into my room an hour later, I was standing quietly beside the bed, wondering how I could climb up into it.

She saw my dilemma right away, and disappeared into the kitchen. She returned with a home-made wooden stool, and when she set it in place, I managed to land in bed after a bit of a roll to protect my broken arm.

When she pulled the covers up over me, it was an awkward moment for both of us. She patted my forehead and said goodnight. I did not know her, and she did not know me. We probably both went to sleep with misgivings. I looked around the shadowy room, everything perfectly tidy. I wondered how long she would keep me.

In 1931, at the time I moved in, the drought had already started. But to a child of my age, that was not a concern. My aunt provided the basics for me, which is all I could have expected. I attended the town school in Cala with our next-door neighbors, known as the Rogers kids. I walked over the train tracks with them each morning for school.

Our teacher, Mr. Peters, was fair and firm. He kept us in line with high expectations in work and play, and his punishments amounted only to being kept in at recess. In later years, I heard about evil teachers who made life unbearable for the particular students they chose to single out. Mr. Peters was a kindly man, which in my case was fortunate, because I had a well-founded fear of men, having been abused by my dad, and sheltered since then by living with my aunt.

On Friday afternoons, our teacher distributed song sheets that were printed on cheap, yellow newsprint, and were huge when we opened them up. We were allowed to sit in pairs, because there weren't enough song sheets to go around. I always sat with Ruth Rogers, and we sang our little hearts out, because we both loved music. Mr. Peters used an annoying pitch pipe to get us started on the right note. They were old songs that I had heard Aunt Flo singing around the house: "Put on Your Old Grey Bonnet", "Bicycle Built for Two", "Little Brown Jug" and others.

The students chose the next song by calling out the number. Every session, one of the boys was sure to call out "Number 12", as it appeared to be a real favorite. Mr. Peters tooted the starting note on his little pipe and everyone sang loudly:

Ha, ha, ha, you and me,
Little brown jug, don't I love thee.

I was horrified when I heard the words. My dad's little brown jug had caused me great pain and sorrow, and so I changed it up. Every time the rest sang "don't I love thee", I nearly yelled out, "don't I **hate** thee!" Mr. Peters never said a word to me about it.

When I started school in September, I was well behind the students my age, but by Christmas Mr. Peters had me reading with the rest in my grade. Aunt Flo found out from him where I was lacking in arithmetic, and she set up multiplication, division, addition, and subtraction cards for me to work on each night after supper. It paid off, and once I met her standard and Mr. Peters was satisfied, I took on additional chores.

Early on, I realized my aunt was not well. She was concerned that I did not strain my arm that had been broken before I arrived. We became a team, even at my young age, looking out for each other. I understood she had taken me in out of the goodness of her heart, and I wanted to be as helpful as possible. Her house was clean, and I felt safe. I never heard directly from my brother. But sometimes a note came in the mail, addressed to my aunt, saying where he was, and asking if we were doing okay.

Aunt Flo had me pedaling the Singer sewing machine when I was barely 11 years old. She started me off hemming the edges of baby diapers that she provided for newborns in the area. She bought used flour sacks at the store for five cents each, and we made stacks of diapers.

She was lavish with her praise, which egged me on to complicated sewing projects. At her insistence, I had become proficient with knitting needles and embroidery thread, but for me, running the machine was exhilarating. There were only a couple of projects I had to rip out and redo. Right away, I could see I was faster than Aunt Flo was when I got to pedaling.

How I envied the farm students who came to our school in town! They had horses, and lived a different lifestyle than we did. I was elated when Mr. Rogers made a deal with my Aunt Flo. He had no feed for his cow, yet he desperately needed milk for his children.

My aunt offered to board the cow at our place, and volunteered me to do the milking. We promised to deliver milk to them each day, and we would use the excess ourselves, or sell it for nine or ten cents a quart. In this way, our neighbors had milk, and the hope of getting the cow back when times were better.

Carl Rogers led their cow over to our yard. She must have thought she had died and gone to heaven as she eyed up the untouched grass at the back of our property. Bally arrived thin and hungry, but deliverance was on the way! My resourceful aunt had various connections for feed, old screenings from the elevator, some hay from up north, and any and all cut up vegetables that could be fed to her. We babied that cow as if she were a princess. It was a joy to behold as we watched her fatten up until her sharp, pointy hip bones were no more.

As a teenager, I dreamed I had achieved farmer status when that big black and white cow joined our flock of chickens! The shed at the back of our property was already housing the chickens and it would be adequate for Bally when shelter was needed. It turned out that she was a very profuse milk producer and my aunt sold numerous nine-cent quarts of milk to folks who needed it.

And so, my early teens were spent at the sewing machine, milking our cow and distributing the milk, and carrying bucket after bucket of water to our pathetic garden. My happiest moments when the work was done, were tearing through the bushes with the Rogers gang.

I attended school until I was 14 years old and received a letter of congratulations from the Department of Education for my achievement—"Completion of Grade 8, With Honors".

By then, I was old enough to realize the severity of the drought. Saskatchewan was burning up! Occasionally, grey clouds rolled in and the wind took on an eerie force. Each time that happened, we rushed outside, hoping against hope that the miracle rains were coming. A few dozen sharp, stinging drops landed at our feet, and that was it. I could imagine the forces of nature sneering, "There. That's all you get!"

After enduring the drought year after year, the farmers lost hope, desperately counting on scant relief support from the government. They took cream, eggs, and butter to the store to trade for flour and sugar. Food was the number one priority.

The ingenuity and work that went into feeding prairie families was nothing short of amazing. Saskatoon bushes in the dry pastures were stripped bare, the berries soaked in cold, salted water to flush out any worms that may have found the bounty before we did. Aunt Flo believed saskatoons were loaded with vitamin C, and so she made sure I didn't overlook any in the ditches or the field behind our yard. The canner was bubbling on our stove throughout the summer.

One spring, we found leftover turnips and carrots in the cellar that had been stored during winter in a bin of sand. We got out the canner and sealers and pickled them before they went soft. We wasted nothing.

Other provinces took pity on us, and throughout the thirties when we needed it most, generous provisions arrived at the train station. Ontario sent huge rounds of cheese, and apples came from British Columbia. Hay and vegetables that could be spared came from Manitoba. The heavily salted cod from Nova Scotia was a puzzle to the prairie folks, and not even resourceful Aunt Flo could come up with a cooking method to make it palatable. One farmer told us he nailed it to the barn door for a salt lick for his cows.

Of course, there were fervent prayers for rain, but the drought persisted. The gardens in town, if they grew at all, were stunted and parched. We carried gallons of water to the scraggly rows near our homes, but it was to no avail. The soil had turned to powder.

It was out of this desperate situation that the idea of a community garden was born, and it proved to be a life-saving inspiration. I believe the thought originated with some of the ladies, but it was the mayor, Frank Hamilton, who made it happen.

The key was water for the plants. Near the train station, right next to the pump house, there were two empty lots which were selected as the ideal location. With Frank Hamilton heading up the plan, the town paid farmers to haul in wagon loads of well-aged manure. (Whoever thought in those days of poverty that the old piles behind the barn could garner a bit of cash?) The soil was prepared with care, and well-watered.

Months previously, the town secretary sent a large order to a well-known seed company down east. The townspeople were asked to bring all leftover potatoes they could spare from their cellars. Most of us had to "sprout our potatoes" a time or two during the winter months to keep them from going soft. This spring, every sprout on the donated seed potatoes was like money in the bank. Some flower seeds, dormant for years, had also been donated. We were thrilled when splashes of color showed up among the rows.

We were young teenagers then, and committed ourselves to the cause, excited to be involved in growing food. We were the faithful water brigade, taking turns at the pump and passing buckets hand to hand. We fooled around a lot, and it became a happy part of our day. That summer, the heat was unbearable, and so we chose to meet in the early mornings or the evenings. Residents from all over town made their way to the community garden after supper, when the wind died down and the heat diminished. Neighbors chatted while they worked with a hoe or a bucket, to the sound of the birds twittering as they put themselves to sleep. There was, and is, nothing that compares with a Saskatchewan sunset at the end of the day. Dirty Thirties or not, the beauty of the prairie sky was unsurpassed. The exception was when the dust clouds were blowing, and the setting sun gave off an eerie orange glow.

The mayor appeared one evening in July and said he needed to talk to us. As we gathered around, he asked if we had noticed the potato bugs. Of course, we had! Hundreds of the hateful, greyish, fat larvae were stuck to the leaves of our thriving potato plants. Frank equipped each of us with a container of kerosene and a stick, and we dealt with them row by row, as we tapped the disgusting, clinging bugs into the deadly liquid.

That summer, we managed a harvest of vegetables to be shared all over town. To celebrate, Frank organized a fall dance with some volunteer musicians, and set up a roaring bonfire. Potatoes were raked out of the coals at the end of the party. They were black and delicious.

Just before it was over, Frank commended the teenagers who had put in so much effort to make the garden a success. I don't know who started it, but in the midst of thanks to the teens, someone yelled, *Fire! Fire! Fire!* The whole crowd burst into the song we sang in Mr. Peter's music class.

> *Late last night when we were all in bed,*
> *Old Lady Leary lit a lantern in the shed.*
> *And when the cow kicked it over,*
> *She winked her eye and said,*
> *There'll be a hot time, in the old town tonight!*
> *Fire! Fire! Fire!*

We were packed like sardines in a circle around the bonfire, and two groups were singing the song as a round. It was a night to remember.

I forget which province sent it, somewhere down east, but the station master arrived one afternoon with what he described as sewing supplies. He loaded the freight on to the wagon, hitched up his team, and made the delivery to our house, as we were known as the seamstresses of the town. He knew my aunt was fair, and would play no favorites in distributing these effects. We were already repairing and replacing worn-out clothes. We patched over patches, and were always scrounging for used clothing that could be revamped.

This new delivery, compliments of John McDonald and his black Clydesdale team, contained six large boxes. We could only imagine how useful this gift was going to be! Before he left, he rather reluctantly produced a pair of his overalls. They were neatly folded and very faded.

"I'm wondering if you might be able to patch the patches on these Sunday go-to-meeting pants of mine. I blew out both knees again." He would pay us a little for our efforts, and we were pleased to do it. He wished us well, and left with a tip of his hat.

I eagerly brought the boxes into our kitchen, and got a butcher knife to open them up. To our wonder and dismay, the box contained rather useless garments from higher society than we were -

girdles, garters, lace jackets, and lingerie. Box after box revealed the same contents. Whoever sent them had no idea of the drudgery and long days our local women put in! They probably thought the items would add some spice to life out west! None of this would be put to any use at all. How disappointing!

My aunt and I continued to work on some items we had been hired to fix up. We charged so little it was pathetic, but we needed to eat too, and my aunt's sewing machine could do wonders.

At exactly three o'clock, Aunt Flo headed for the kitchen to put the kettle on for tea. No matter the day, or the lack of resources, we had tea at three every afternoon, rain or shine! (Cancel that, there was no rain!)

I grabbed John's overalls, and I slid into my place in front of the Singer machine. It didn't take long to reinforce the old patches and sew on larger new ones. We had a pile of old clothing, and pieces of fabric that were as precious as gold when we tackled our sewing jobs, especially repair jobs like this.

As I finished, I had a brainwave. It was silly, to be sure, but one of the fancy girdles was sticking out of the opened box, and I spied a couple of bright red bows just waiting to be put to use. I sewed them by hand with tight stitches to John McDonald's overalls at the same time as my aunt called me to the table for tea.

I placed my work on the table and my aunt, usually of a serious nature, burst into giggles at the sight of red satin on the bib of the overalls. Of course, that was followed by my loud "Liz laugh" as we both, no doubt, imagined him going around town in ribbons and bows. When I turned the garment over, she could see I had also sewn an even bigger bow to the rear. I could tell my aunt's laughter had turned to tears as she said, "It shows how desperate we are just for a laugh."

We had our tea with milk stirred into it, and then headed for the train station, not far from our house. We immediately saw his team still tied to the hitching post outside the station. John was sitting on the well-used bench by the wall where the townspeople, young and old, waited for the train to come in each evening. He had a torn, red handkerchief in his hand, mopping his forehead.

I handed over the carefully folded overalls and proclaimed with a flourish, "Parker and Melbourne Seamstress Company at your service, and delivered to your door!"

He shook out the pants and immediately saw the bow on the backside. It started with a slight shaking of his shoulders. Then his face turned bright red, and finally, he lifted his chin off his chest and roared out a laugh that could be heard across town.

"You know you're not getting these ribbons back! I'm going to wear them with pride, and I'll have the admiration of the whole community."

We refused payment when he offered it, as we had already received more than we put into that afternoon effort. By the next morning, an ingenious plan had taken shape in my aunt's mind.

Our girls' sewing class, age ten and up, would take on new lessons, that of salvage. Our weekly Saturday afternoons would, for the next while at least, involve careful stitch ripping, to provide us with lace, elastic, and ribbons. What a treasure trove of notions for future sewing projects! Every baby layette, which we often worked on with the girls, would be trimmed with something special. Girls and ladies would have the luxury of pretty trim added to their sadly worn clothing.

My aunt said it brought to mind the adage, "Never look a gift horse in the mouth". When I asked her for the meaning, she explained a horse's teeth reveal its age. So, if a horse is received as a gift, don't be looking in its mouth to check whether it's a young, valuable horse. I caught on right away.

"I get it, Aunt Flo, we'll just say thank you for the fripperies from down east, and put them to the best possible use." I was reminded of the salted cod, sent to us by caring Nova Scotians. It is true, we should never look a gift horse in the mouth.

Aunt Flo fairly distributed community donations to those in need, but she did personally take on the Wilson family after they lost their three-year-old boy. It was heartbreaking that children in the province were suffering from malnutrition, and many of them had rickets. She got us a ride out to Wilson's farm one Sunday afternoon. The memory of that visit has never left me.

We came bearing gifts. I thought, as we packed the buggy and left our house, that she was being a little excessive taking this and that from various rooms of our house. She had me stand on a chair and hand down the contents of a storage cupboard above her bedroom clothes closet. There were various odds and sods, some special dishes, cushions, glass cups, doilies, a couple of framed scenic photos. I wondered what the Wilsons would want with Aunt Flo's stored keepsakes.

When I entered their house and realized their destitution, I understood. Any bit of anything was welcome and needed. Practical, matter-of-fact Aunt Flo had no time for sentiment that day. She had me unload the boxes from the buggy, and carry them into the house.

She began with the food. She unpacked every item as the children gathered around and gazed with wonder at sealers of rhubarb and saskatoons, and one of canned chicken, a loaf of fresh bread, a jar of soup, potatoes, and cabbage from our sparse garden, and two quilts we had made "for a rainy day". Well, rainy days didn't happen, and so it was only sensible to pass them on to these folks who had the barest house I had ever seen.

My aunt momentarily took over their home, pointing at the broom, indicating I was to give the floor a thorough sweeping. As I did, the children continued to gape at Aunt Flo. She spread out the bounty: the doilies, a braided rag rug by the door, quilts smoothed flat, one on each of the two beds, dishes added to the cupboard, cups upside down as we all did in those days to keep out the dust. I was amazed and thrilled to see how perfectly each offering enhanced that dreary home. It took on a look of hope and promise. The oldest boy was sent for a hammer, and wise as ever, Aunt Flo had a couple of nails in her pocket. With supervision, the boy hung the pictures by the window.

We brought along clothes for the kids. We had guessed at their sizes as we busied ourselves at the trusty Singer the previous week. It wouldn't matter if they fit just right or not, we knew they'd wear whatever we brought.

Before we left, I saw my aunt slip her arm around Mrs. Wilson's back and promise two quarts of milk per week, and diapers, and a layette for the upcoming baby. Mrs. Wilson, a woman of few words, responded with a faint smile. Placing her arm across her bulging midsection she said, "I think this one is another boy."

Mr. Wilson appeared from outside and glanced around the room. He clasped my aunt's right hand and pumped it up and down to show his gratefulness.

"You are angels," he said. "Angels sent straight from heaven."

I noticed he said "angels", plural. I was included, even though I had done practically nothing, besides carrying the boxes and sweeping the floor.

After that visit, along with the milk we gave each week, we included something extra to eat, usually a jar of soup. My aunt was clever and creative. "Make something out of nothing" was her motto.

When I used the very last of the apples Aunt Betty shipped to us by train from BC, I peeled them ever so carefully and made a special dessert. I proudly placed it on the table for a special afternoon tea, and announced, "It's an apple brown betty in honor of Aunt Betty's gift." My aunt looked at me rather apologetically and said, "Do you think we might save it for the Wilsons?"

A wish-to-be-forgotten day started with a bunch of us venturing out in the pasture south of town to pick chokecherries. Not much of anything would grow during the dry years, as even the hardy poplar trees had died, or were dying from lack of rain. But there were chokecherries, and we had hopes of jelly or jam preserves to improve pancakes and bread.

With a full bucket or two delivered to each of our homes, we were still looking for some fun, and tree climbing was a long-standing pastime. There were some tall trees where the creek used to run, and so we monkeyed our way up the tallest of them, trying out different trees to see who could climb the highest.

Minutes after we started, we all heard a deafening crack as one of the dry tree trunks snapped under Carl's weight. He fell down the side of the tree grasping for a handhold as he went. Near the bottom, in his descent, he sort-of bounced against the trunk, and then landed on his back. An ugly sight visited my dreams for weeks after. Carl's eye. It must have caught the sharp stump of a branch on his way down.

I later said to my aunt, "Of all the places on his body, why his eye!"

She said, in her practical way, "Better his eye than his heart."

There was blood and screaming, and my long legs took me swiftly to the center of town. The elderly doctor grabbed his bicycle from the side of his house and pedaled furiously to keep up with me. I led him through Main Street and over the grassy path back to Carl. Carl's sister Ruth left the scene when I did, and lagged behind me, but by the time I returned with the doctor, she had alerted her mother. They, too, were speeding to the tall trees by the old creek bed.

Carl wore a patch on his eye for a long while after his stay in the hospital in Stillwater, and was later fitted with a glass eye. It probably changed his life in more ways than he knew. For one thing, when the boys from the area joined up for the war, he was turned down for military duty.

A tragedy like Carl's eye injury strengthens the bonds of friendship. After that awful day, Ruth, Carl, and I spent increased time together, and it was about that time in our early teens that we grew out of our childish games and moved on to getting jobs and taking on added responsibility.

Those memories were as clear to me as if they had happened yesterday. I spent much of my time at the hospital mulling over my growing up years. I had one foot in the past, and one in the present. In Cala, I had been surrounded by people I loved, and people who loved me. That was the difference. Here, no one cared if I lived or died, at least that's how it felt to me most of the time.

DIG DEEP!

As time went by, I garnered additional information about the hospital. Some of it I would rather not have known, while other details were fascinating. I still wondered who was running the show. It was a vast place, with countless patients and staff to organize and to keep on task. There was an entire area called "Shacktown", comprised of housing for staff who were living on the grounds. The cluster of buildings included a school for their children. Those families shared our space, almost as if we all were citizens of a private city.

The site for the hospital had been chosen specifically for its scenic and peaceful location on the edge of the woodland. No doubt, the river view was refreshing for our souls.

We were offered meaningful work. Some patients were exhausted from overwork, but were determined to comply. Some refused to move, and sat staring at the wall, lost in dark depression. Screaming in the night was unnerving, and it set off alarm bells in my mind. What was happening to those women I could hear calling out in the Women's Ward, crying, moaning, shrieking? It didn't happen all the time. I know there was mistreatment of some of the patients, as I heard about it directly from them, and I believed what they told me. I was never abused in any way. My condition did not call for experimental treatments that were forced on mentally ill patients at that time.

Lily kept me informed with her version of what was going on. One day, out of the blue, she said, "I listen to the nurses, you know. They hate the insulin shock treatments." I had heard about insulin injections that eventually caused convulsions and comas, apparently in an attempt to cure schizophrenia. Though I had no concrete information, I did know that I agreed with the nurses.

The overcrowding was an increasing issue. The huge population represented thousands of needs. Human beings were smothered with feelings of loneliness and abandonment. For most, it was a dark place, and for some, merely an existence. Despite the barriers, mental health treatment was slowly progressing. There were doctors like Dr. Sanders who were eager to explore the field and discover improvements.

Speaking of Dr. Sanders, he did not mention the plan for "outpatients" again. Perhaps the war had slowed progress in that area, or he had lost the dream. I was a minuscule cog in a huge wheel. I was practically invisible in the big scheme of things, and no one from the outside was breaking down the door to find me. I pushed away the notion of being discharged, because I understood myself well. If I counted on being released, the longing to get out would swallow me up.

I looked around to discover my best recourse. I am sorry for folks who didn't have an Aunt Flo. Her wise words came to me when I needed them most. "Dig deep and you will find something, not for yourself, but something to give someone else." I remembered that advice when I began assisting the nurses with the elderly patients. I made a promise to myself that I would try to bring some light and love to the loneliest people around me. Even when there was no visible response, I felt better for trying.

Staff members encouraged me to learn new skills. Little did I know, the hospital had a canteen and post office! Also, up and running, were cabinet making, carpentry, toy making, shoe repair, dry-cleaning - you name it! The opportunities for me to learn were endless, and unlike when I arrived, I was now allowed my choice of where I would work, and when.

A patient named Ewald enjoyed his work in the woodworking shop. I worked there too for six months, and learned about different tools, and how to use them. With direction from our supervisor, Ewald and I each made a crude cribbage board, carefully drilling holes with what was called an eggbeater drill, using the various sized bits stored in the handle. We used matchsticks for markers, and for several weeks, noon hours for us included a game of crib.

I took some lessons in the beauty parlor and barbershop. The main barber there said I had a knack for it, and invited me to help at any time. From the time I was a kid, my aunt had encouraged me to accumulate all the skills possible, as they would come in handy. She had insisted on the sewing and handwork, as well as housekeeping, cooking, and baking.

She admired my ability to milk our cow, and she often commented on it, perhaps because she had never milked a cow herself. I assured her I found it rather satisfying. Bally was a docile old girl and the strong and steady streams of milk hitting the bottom of the tin milk pail were music to my ears.

Things were slowly changing at the hospital. Those changes were for the better, and are probably what carried me through the following years. I spent time with people, both staff and patients, and I found ways to "dig deep", as my aunt had told me to.

OUTPATIENT

O n July 18th, my 28th birthday, I received the best gift I could have imagined. I was washing windows in the bedridden ladies' room, using newspaper and vinegar water, as I had been taught long ago. The windows were sparkling, and I had only one left to go, when suddenly, I noticed Marj standing in the doorway with a huge grin on her face. The thought flashed through my mind that she may have known it was my birthday. I dried my hands on the skirt of my dress and went to meet her.

Suddenly and unexpectedly, Marj was crying and laughing at the same time. Obviously choked up, she spoke anyway, her freckles standing out on her red face.

"Liz, I've wanted this day to come for years. Finally, I'm allowed to invite you to come home with me, and live at my house!"

Stunned is the best word to describe my reaction. I know my eyebrows went straight up, signaling a million questions.

Marj stretched out her hands in front of her, palms up. "It's the Outpatients Program - at last!"

"Really?" I burst out laughing. I did a fancy little dance, as Marj dried her tears, and my trademark belly laugh echoed down the hallway.

"When?"

"Whenever we want."

"How about right now!" I was yelling, but I didn't care.

It was Marj's day off, and she had already signed the papers taking responsibility for me under the Outpatients Program. The arrangement was exactly as Dr. Sanders had outlined years ago. Marj would be paid a stipend for my room and board, and for helping me ease back into the community. I would be expected to eventually find a job and make my way, but in the meantime, I would work part-time as a volunteer at the hospital. I was also expected to behave myself. It was an experiment, and Marj and I were determined to make it a success.

She insisted on taking me to a Chinese restaurant for ice cream on the way home, to celebrate my status as an outpatient. While we were enjoying the strawberry ice cream, served in a metal pedestal dish lined with cone-shaped paper, I told her it was my birthday. Tears instantly came to her eyes.

"This is meant to be, Liz."

Marj was single. She drove an old model car that was beat-up on the outside, but she said it ran well enough to get her across the river for work, and that was all she needed.

Her house was not stylish in any way, but it was homey and welcoming. She showed me my room. Oh, it had been years since I had my own room! A bed, a dresser, a braided rug on the floor. And blessings of all blessings, a little Philco radio on a bedside table. Music made my world go round, and I had missed having it at my fingertips since leaving Aunt Flo's house. I was giddy and trying to rein myself in. Marj noticed, and told me just to be myself.

"I like who you are, Liz. We are going to do fine!"

The next day, we drove around the city. Marj said it was so I could "get my bearings". I had become familiar with the city of Stillwater when I worked at the Aviation School café. As we drove past the airfield, she commented that the training school had closed down in '44.

We went to the grocery store, and she encouraged me to select foods I preferred. Years ago, I did all the shopping for my aunt and me. I was fascinated with the new foods offered, and the different packaging on the shelves.

The storekeeper rang up our rather large order on an adding machine, and packed the items in a cardboard box. Marj paid for the groceries, and I carried them to the car. Teamwork. I knew grocery shopping would once again become an ordinary event, but this time it was a strange mix of novel and familiar at the same time.

Marj gave me a printed paper to read with the heading, "Outpatient Program". Four goals were listed:

1. Ease the patient back into the world of normal living
2. Assist with social adjustment
3. Engage in meaningful work or hobbies
4. Encourage friends and family to visit

Marj said she and other home providers had attended a couple of meetings discussing the goals. I suggested that even our grocery shopping had to do with number 1. She agreed. We talked about social adjustment. Marj's friends, who came over every week to play cards, were eager to meet me.

I expressed my desire to find work right away, and get back into the swing of things. Marj knew I had worked at the Air Training School café, and already had an idea where I could work. It happened that the coffee shop down the street was looking for an employee. The hours were nine to two, as they served only breakfast and lunch, catering to the working crowd. They specialized in fresh coffee, bacon and eggs, and pancakes. Lunch was sandwiches and pie. As soon as I heard about the vacancy, I wanted that job so I could prove myself.

As to the fourth goal, I knew how I wanted to deal with it. I told my host that I would very soon write a letter to my brother Ralph and request a meeting, as we had some business to settle. She suggested that as time passed, she and I could take a drive around my former town, and perhaps renew old acquaintances. We were excited, and on the same page.

BUCK'S DINER

Marj went with me to the coffee shop to meet the boss. He was a big man with a mustache, and went by the nickname, Buck. I got the job easily. I believe I was hired on the reliable name of my host, who was well known in the community, and admired for who she was.

I handled the workload with ease. In fact, it was nothing compared to an exhausting full day's work in the hot kitchens at the hospital. This shift was only five hours. It went fast, with lots of customers coming and going, especially during the noon rush hour.

I was trained by the boss, who wore a stiff, white apron and was very particular about handwashing, and running a sanitary kitchen. He showed me where the supplies were stored, and we worked together making sandwiches ahead of the lunch hour. The coffee machine was constantly running - no wonder the shop was known for quality, fresh coffee. We moved smoothly through the morning, clearing tables, washing dishes, and serving customers. A McGavins truck delivered several flats of bread each day at ten o'clock, to be kept in the cool room at the back of the shop. I was getting the hang of the place, relieved to see it was a very pleasant job that would help me regain a comfort level with people on the outside.

Buck was known for calling all ladies by his pet name for them, "Gorgeous." He left out the "r" so we were all "Goh-jus", whether it was Helen (the other employee) or me, or any female customer who came in. He was a great boss, and expected nothing of us that he wouldn't do himself. He worked alone after two o'clock, when he washed the place down, bleached the floors, and made pies for the next day.

I was told that Helen worked on Fridays and the weekends. After a week of training, I was surprised to see Helen already inside the shop when I went in for my first shift on my own. She said Buck had asked her to come in to make sure I got through the day alright.

"Hi, I'm Liz." I extended my hand, and she shook it without much enthusiasm. She didn't offer her name.

As she was tying on her apron, she looked at me with sort of a sneer and said, "I know what we'll do. You can be Popeye, I'll be Olive and we can serve spinach sandwiches!"

I don't believe in tattle-tales, nor have I ever been one, but at that moment, I did what I had to do. I went to the dial phone in the kitchen and called Marj. She was home from work that morning, and I simply asked if she could come. She walked through the door in about five minutes, and waited for me to tell her what was going on. Helen pretended to wipe off the kitchen counter. I didn't care that she was listening.

"Marj, thanks for coming. I'm sorry to bother you, but I know you are responsible for me and how things are going at my job. Helen here has insulted me, and I don't know what we should do about it."

Without making eye contact, Helen spoke up. "I was joking. Can't you take a joke?"

I repeated to Marj what Helen had said. I felt like a kid in school, tattling to the teacher. Maybe I should have let it go.

Marj was perturbed. "That is downright nasty, Helen. You well know Liz is on her first job after being in the Saskatchewan hospital. She's right in saying I am responsible for her. I'll have to talk to Buck, and see what he wants to do about this."

Helen was ready to back down. "Buck's been praising her work to high heaven since the day she started. I need this job, I really do!"

I heard a voice in the back of my head. Aunt Flo again, teaching me how to live right. "Liz, if someone is going to be mean, make sure it's not you!"

I wanted to do the right thing. "I'll tell you what, Helen. We could start this day over again. I don't think Buck needs to hear about this. He's a busy guy."

Helen nodded. I was pretty sure things were settled. I hoped so, anyway.

"Thanks, Marj, for coming. I'm okay."

We had an agreeable shift together. Helen was an efficient worker, and because there were two of us, we had extra time before the lunch crowd came in. We took a couple of minutes for a break, chatting in the kitchen.

I believe in being direct, so I said, "I want to tell you about my eyes."

"No, please, it's okay."

"Well, just so you know, it's not catchy! It's a thyroid thing that I'm stuck with."

I told Marj about that conversation, and she commended me for clearing the air. "People react better when they understand. You did the right thing today, Liz." Marj was endeavoring to be an exceptional home provider in the Outpatient Program. She would likely record the day's events, and report them at their meeting, which was fine with me.

The novelty of normal living was invigorating. I loved cooking and baking in Marj's kitchen, cleaning the house, and washing clothes. It was all giving me a sense that I was the same person I used to be. Marj was, for some reason, surprised that I could cook. She appreciated having supper on the table when she returned from her work across the river. "I'm already fat enough, and if you cook like this, I'm in trouble!"

MY BROTHER RALPH

I wrote my letter to Ralph, and wondered what his response would be. I told him I was living at an outpatient placement and he could visit me here at this address, not at the hospital. I had intended it to be a warm letter, starting on the right foot again, but I wasn't able to word it that way. I point blank asked for the money I had entrusted to him, and I asked him to bring my little girl to see me.

I contemplated my history with my brother. In truth, I hardly knew him. I was born when he was ten years old, and soon after that, he was spending as much time as he could elsewhere. Marj asked how I felt about his hoped-for visit after all these years. I shared with her the story of Ralph Parker, at least my version of it.

Ralph had taken his share of abuse from our father, as I had, so rather than help on the farm when local jobs ran out, he hit the road. He placed me safely at Aunt Flo's, and became a hobo like thousands of other single young men in the 1930s. They could hardly be called men. Rather, they were boys who had dropped out of school to "work out", so as not to be a burden at home. There were thousands of them across the country, who weren't allotted government relief. Ralph knew how to work. Our dad had seen to that, but no one could afford to hire. Jobs had dried up, due to the dust and drought.

He wrote from time to time to Aunt Flo, and she read his letters out loud to me. She had a soft spot in her heart for her brother's two motherless children. I would guess she sent Ralph a little money from time to time, although she truly had none to spare.

Ralph ended up working in a bush camp in British Columbia, sponsored by the Department of National Defense, where they built roads, cleared brush, and planted trees. The men were aware it was busywork, and their resentment grew. They were given food, a place to sleep, and 20 cents a day for their efforts. From rumors we heard about those construction camps, conditions were rough and primitive, and hundreds of restless men felt like cattle in a holding corral. They wished, as we all did, for life to go back to normal, where honest work paid off and a man could get ahead, if he wasn't lazy.

Ralph wrote that he longed for a future where he could settle down, marry the French girl he had met in northern Saskatchewan, and have a family. Sometimes, he wrote long letters to Aunt Flo about his hopes and plans, but as time went on his communications became shorter. Finally, he sent only a postcard now and then, hardly worth the three-cent stamp.

His notes assured us he was alive. Many of the hobos who took to the rails were not. It was dangerous business, jumping off and on the boxcars and ducking the railway guards who were hired to get rid of them. Sometimes, a photo of hundreds of men riding on top of the train appeared in the newspaper, their faces black and eyes swollen from the smoke and the cinders. It was not first-class transportation by any means.

One of Ralph's postcards merely contained these words: "April, 1935. Walked out of camp. Taking the rails to Vancouver".

My aunt ate up every word published in the paper. The men from the relief camp congregated in Vancouver, as a public challenge to the government to come up with decent jobs for a fair wage. They were orderly and persistent, but made no progress in obtaining work. Ralph's next postcard simply read, "Ottawa or bust". Aunt Flo had a hunch it would not end well.

The trekkers were heading east, where they planned to demand justice from the federal government. As it turned out, they didn't make it past Regina, and Aunt Flo's hunch proved true. Prime Minister Bennett decreed they be stopped in Regina. On orders from Ottawa, the RCMP stormed an orderly strikers' meeting, arrested the leaders, and the battle was on! Known ever after as the Regina Riot, the confrontation on July 1 with RCMP, city police, citizens of the city, and the trekkers continued for hours. Cars were shoved into the streets as barricades. RCMP were forced off their horses. It was called a pitch battle, involving rocks, bricks, bottles, tear gas, and guns, and resulted in two deaths, untold injuries, and costly damage to the city.

We heard the news of it the next day, but no word on Ralph. In the wee small hours of the morning, I found my aunt sitting on our porch, huddled in a blanket, worrying over her nephew. I realized then how much she cared about my brother and me, and how fortunate we were to have her devotion.

Five days later, another postcard arrived. I can still see my aunt frantically scanning the note. She closed her eyes with a sigh of relief as his few words sunk in. "Things turned bloody in Regina. Stayed out of it. Back in camp. RP". The camp closed down the following year, and luckily for my brother, the farm was available to him that spring when Dad died.

I was almost 13 when we got word of my dad's death. I felt nothing good or bad towards him. My aunt had talked me through the situation more than once. She said he was the one who lost out, and we should feel sorry for him. Being a fighter, I carried some anger that he used his size and power against me, and I had entertained little girl thoughts of going back there to settle the score. In my heart, I realized my aunt was right. He was a pathetic, needy man who squandered not only his livelihood, but his children.

She offered to take me to the funeral, but I opted to stay home, as I had no desire to go back there. I told her I would oversee the ranch, even though our "ranch" consisted of one cow and a few old laying hens. I suppose my refusal showed I had not yet come to terms with my father's abuse.

Aunt Flo's sister, Betty, came from BC and they were gone for a week, attending to their brother's affairs. When she returned, she gave me a framed photo of my parents' wedding day, and a small picture of me as a baby, sitting on Ralph's knee. At ten years old, he looked proud as punch of his baby sister.

Ralph's inheritance was more substantial than mine. It was very convenient for him at that time to step up and take ownership of the farm, as it provided a much-needed home for him and his wife, Irene. Aunt Flo said the farm was in deplorable condition, and the house barely livable, but she hoped the young couple could make a go of it, despite the drought. At last, Ralph had a place to hang his hat, which gave my aunt as much relief as if he had been her own son.

Marj was fascinated with Ralph's story. She pointed out the positives she had noted from my account, and suggested I make an effort to include him in my life.

ROOM FOR ONE MORE

I was delighted to be living with Marj, and she was so enthused with the arrangement that she requested a second patient to join us. When she brought it up, I wondered how that would work, but she had thought it through. She said I had the final say, as she did not want to jeopardize the close relationship we were building.

Marj's house had two bedrooms, and I was hoping I wouldn't have to give up the privilege of having my own room. That remained one of the most luxurious treats of my being out: the privacy, sleeping alone, no yelling, no snoring, at least no snoring by others!

Her idea was brilliant. She offered me her sun porch. It was a room with windows that ran the width of the house, a long and narrow, bright room that I already favored for Saturday afternoon reading. She shared her intention to paint the walls, and to add a bed, dresser, and some comfortable chairs. There were blinds on the windows for privacy, and she had plans to winterize the room. And so, I happily moved out of the tiny bedroom to make room for our anticipated guest, and settled into a more spacious area. By this time, Buck had paid my first wages and I bought a Philco radio of my own for my room.

I had one slip-up at work, if you could call it that. As I became more comfortable with the customers, I began to enjoy the conversation and interaction. One morning, a new face appeared in the coffee line-up. A crooked grin, and a cap pulled down to his eyebrows. That's what I noticed first. As I approached his table and poured a cup of coffee for him, he said loudly for all to hear, "Hi Smiley!"

I stopped, the world stopped, and for a second I couldn't breathe. That was Ray's name for me. I turned away, and rushed to the back room. Standing there, inhaling the smell of fresh McGavin's bread, I gulped in air, my chest heaving. It only took a second or two. I was okay.

I returned to the confused newcomer who looked at me closely. He asked quietly, "Is something wrong?"

"Nope, everything's fine!"

Everything *was* fine! I had been caught off guard. Just for a moment I experienced a trigger from the past, and it had overwhelmed me, but I had quickly shaken it off. I had vowed to forget that era, but it had popped up right in my face by surprise. I added extra whipped cream to the piece of pie he ordered.

That night I told Marj about it, the sudden unexpected feelings, and my quick recovery.

"I'm glad you told me, Liz. It helps to talk. It seems once we share it, then it really is okay." Her comment was a contrast to the rule of law at the Home for Unwed Mothers. Marj had just said it helps to talk. There they forbade us to talk, either then or later. We were expected to bottle up our shameful secret, and never speak of it again.

I thought of the number one goal of the outpatient program, "Ease the patient back into normal living". I was easing in all right, happy to be where I was, looking hopefully toward a fulfilling future. I volunteered at the hospital two days a week. It was becoming harder and harder to believe that I had lived there for years. I felt comfortable on the outside, and I was not all that eager to go back for my volunteer hours. The nurses appreciated my help feeding and working with the old ladies, but the main push was that I, along with some of the other outpatients, would put our energies into helping with a knitting club and music therapy. These programs were in the beginning stages, and overall, I enjoyed helping out.

Lily quickly approached me on my visit back to the hospital. She was on the gardening crew, flitting as usual from place to place, chatting with whoever would listen.

"The nurses call you the Outpatient. Do you like that?"

"Yes, I do."

"Well, I'm the Inpatient. It's best for me."

"You are a top-notch Inpatient, Lily. I will never forget when you came and talked to me when I was sad. You helped me."

She burst out laughing, and said, "I knew you were sad."

I invited her to the music club, and I asked if I should come and get her when it was time to start. She squinted her eyes for a moment and then said, "I sing better than you. I better come."

She rushed to meet me on another afternoon when I arrived for my knitting class. Looking one way and then the other, she whispered, "Did you hear about the 'crippler'?" She was referring to polio, the terrifying epidemic that had started in the late '40s but had come on even stronger in the 1950s. Lily looked at me mysteriously, as if deciding whether or not to divulge a secret.

"Some of them are here now. Did you know?"

I did know. They had found refuge in the hospital, as their families were not equipped to care for them at home. I was counting on the volunteers to seek them out, and offer hope and friendship.

I thought about them that evening, as I washed the dishes. Life can change so swiftly, as it had for the polio victims, mowed down by the crippler. One day a person is well and taking life for granted, but within hours or even minutes, the future can be altered and never the same again. The war had also forever changed families, stealing sons and brothers like a thief in the night. And of course, I had firsthand knowledge of how it felt to land in the hospital, my future drastically different than it might have been. Ever on my mind was the fact that a baby born outside of marriage changed the future for so many girls, stuck in the homes for unwed mothers.

THE DIRTY SECRET

That night I told Marj about my pregnancy, and the treatment I received at the Home. For years, I had wanted to talk to someone about it, to tell my "dirty secret" at last, and get it out in the open. I hoped to find freedom from the shame of it, once and for all. Marj was non-judgmental. In fact, she was already familiar with the Home I had been in. Her younger sister, Ellen, had been at the same one.

"I need to talk about it, Marj. Are you up for a long-winded story?"

"Yes, I am, Liz. I have broad shoulders and a listening ear." So, we sat on the couch and drank two pots of tea and I told her the whole story, from start to finish.

"They laid into me minutes after I arrived. From the moment I wrote on their form that I would be taking my baby home with me, the fight was on. I was ridiculed, told I was neurotic, and that I was an unfit mother. They said my pregnancy was proof of that. They drilled into me that I was selfish and foolish. Their main lever was to say that keeping my child as an "illegitimate" took away any chance the baby had to live a respectable life. Oh, Marj, that was a dark place!"

"I know. When Ellen came home, she told me all about it, but neither of us has mentioned it for years."

According to Marj, Ellen had experienced the same coercion. When she agreed to relinquish her baby, they made her swear an oath not to try to find him, ever. They said if she had any care at all for her child, she would leave him alone. I had been on that same path. They tried to break me. More than once, I was sent to the "thinking room" after a bout of arguing with the staff about keeping my baby.

When I explained to Marj that Ralph had my little girl, she put her arm around me, and her eyes filled with tears.

"I had no idea when you came to the hospital what all you were carrying. I was told about the Graves' disease, and I could see you were hurting. I wondered if there may be a hidden secret somewhere behind those big eyes of yours."

I asked Marj about her sister, how she got on after adopting her baby out. "She got married a couple of years later, but she has never told her husband. I am sure no one knows to this day, except my mother and me. Ellen was loud and fun-loving before, but she came out of there very subdued. I think she still suffers depression over what happened. They told her every day, 'When you leave here, forget it ever happened.' I guess that's what she's done. She's buried her secrets. It's heartbreaking that they sent her home to live a lie for the rest of her life."

"I'm sorry about your sister, and I ache for the girls who are there right now."

The hour had grown late. Marj had to work in the morning, but she was unconcerned when I mentioned she needed her rest.

"What happened to you should never have happened, Liz."

Those simple words brought comfort. I had never been offered empathy or compassion about my ordeal until this night. Marj was right - she had broad shoulders and a listening ear.

"You are a beautiful woman Liz, inside and out. Don't let those ugly little voices in your head tell you any different."

I felt lighter. An enormous sense of relief settled over me, as I went to my bedroom. I had not foisted my burden onto Marj, no, far from that! Somehow, in sharing the heaviness that I carried, it had dissolved and disappeared. At that moment, it was even okay that Ralph had my girl. She was safe and cared for, and I would have the privilege of knowing a little of her life and her future as it unfolded.

I pulled the patchwork quilt around my shoulders. I would sleep in peace, unhindered by tangled dreams about my walk of shame at the Home. As I drifted off, I thanked the Lord above for my cherished friend Marj. I remembered Dr. Sander's comment from so many years ago: *A friend is a good thing to have.* He was right about that. Marj was a true friend, who had listened to my heart and had not condemned me.

A VISITOR

On a sunny Saturday in September, Marj and I tackled winterizing the sunroom. We replaced the screens with storm windows that had been stored in the crooked little shed on the east side of the house. We washed and polished them, and after they were in place, we cut strips of cloth to wedge along the window frames to block out the draft. We stuffed in the strips with a table knife, and we did an efficient job. It was a breezy day, so we kept putting our hands on the areas we had already plugged, as a test to see if it was keeping out the wind. There was probably a product at the store to seal the windows, but both Marj and I had learned to pinch pennies during the Dirty '30s. We had several tricks up our sleeves to save money and do it in the old-fashioned way. We agreed that she would have to invest in a storm door to combat the winter chill.

Marj told some of her friends that I was an accomplished seamstress, and I was offered sewing jobs to do in my spare time. I eagerly took them on. Marj had regular customers too, and it felt like old times, sewing as I had on piece work with Aunt Flo, just to make a little more to stretch the budget.

Of course, my immediate project was buying shoes, and sewing clothes for myself when I left the hospital. I preferred to order from the catalogue, as I wasn't ready yet to be a customer in a clothing store. I ordered socks, comfortable, sturdy shoes for work, and fabric to make myself some dresses. Ordering and buying needed items were normal, everyday tasks for normal, everyday people. I felt like I had been a castaway on a far-flung island for a long time.

That afternoon, when our project was complete, the windows were shining, and I curled up in the armchair to read a book. I was happy with the fresh and clean look of the sunroom.

Marj delegated me to choose the color for the paint, and I had surprised her by painting the walls a bright yellow while she was at work. We added some blooming African violets and geraniums. Marj offered a couple of framed pictures of faraway places. I was feeling as content as a cat, when there was a tap on the sunroom door. Finally, Ralph had come.

Our meeting was a bit awkward. I offered him my chair, as it was the most comfortable in the room and I took another. I pulled it up close to him, and always the talker, I began, rather tactlessly, "Did you bring my money?"

"I sure did!" He placed the long, fat envelope in my hand. I half opened it, so I could peek inside. I could tell it hadn't been disturbed.

"You didn't steal a penny from me, Ralph."

"Of course not. There's $20 more in it than there was before. The Home mailed it to me."

"Huh. I'm surprised. I wish they could give back all they took."

My words hung in the air. There was no answer to that. I picked up the conversation, as I assumed Ralph wouldn't.

"So - how long did aunt Flo last in BC?"

"Not long. Just long enough to save your life."

"I think it was *you* who saved me at the Home, that day when the ambulance came."

"No, it was Aunt Flo all the way. She phoned me the night before, and told me she had a hunch."

"Oh, I remember all about her hunches. When she had a hunch, we had to do something about it. It didn't happen often, but she was never wrong."

"She tried to call the Home for weeks, and they refused to let her speak to you. So, she kept phoning me every day, trying to find out if you were okay. That last night when she phoned, there was no getting around it. She said she had a hunch that it was life or death for you. She ordered me to get in my car and drive there, and not waste another minute.

"Irene was livid, as it was late at night and she didn't want me to go. It was snowing, the end of November…"

"Yeah, what day was it?"

"November 29."

"Is that the baby's birthday?"

"Yes."

"So, Aunt Flo knew."

"She sure did. I drove most of the night, as the roads were bad, and I could only go 35 miles an hour from our farm to the city. In the morning, I had breakfast at a coffee shop near the address of the Home, but I kept hearing her urgent order: I've got a hunch, Ralph, and when I get a hunch!"

"The rules stated no one was allowed in there until after 12 noon, but as you may recall, I pounded on the door and finally got an answer."

"And there I was - strange I was right there by the door - I hardly knew where I was."

"You were dying, Sis."

I closed my eyes, seeing my little aunt holding the phone to her ear, bossing Ralph like he was a little kid.

Ralph opened his wallet. "She died soon after that." He handed me a newspaper clipping, an obituary actually, from the *Penticton Herald*, dated December 1944. Her picture was beside the title "Ever Remembered".

"Everything happened so fast that day, Liz. You were right out of it. They did emergency surgery so you could breathe. They deemed you incompetent. When they asked for next of kin, I stepped up, along with that little devil of a director. I was in no mood to deal with her.

"I said, 'Back off lady, I've already been to the police, and they're investigating your care of my sister.' She disappeared, and I signed for the baby. That's how it happened, Sis. I know it's not fair, and it's not right, but I had no choice."

I longed to see her. "You couldn't bring her today?"

"She's only eight. I'm going to tell her though, when she's a little older. I don't believe in secrets."

"Neither do I, but that's what they thrived on at the Home where you dropped me off. Oh, that was a place and a half, Ralph!"

"I know. I saw it with my own eyes. You've had a rough go - the Home, the Graves', the hospital."

We went silent. There was not much to say. I smiled at my big brother. "Life didn't go as we hoped." There was a long pause.

"So, she's eight?"

"Yeah, the same age you were the day I found you in the dirt."

Ralph had described it to me, long before. He was 18 years old, coming home for the weekend, after working away all week. First, he saw a stick with blood on it, then he saw me not making a sound, knocked out.

"What's her name?"

"Marie Jeannette. Irene named her after her mother."

"You could have named her Elizabeth Rose."

"I know. I wanted to."

My six-foot-three brother who took part in the Regina Riot - and proud of it - was a pansy under the harsh thumb of his wife. She called the shots, and my take on that was this. Ralph never wanted to be an abusive brute like our dad. So, he was a pushover when it came to Irene.

"When you tell her, what will you say?"

"I'll tell her you've been ill, and what you have."

"Fair enough."

"What's she like?"

"She's the best kid! She's cute and fun, and she's little for her age."

I remembered Dr. Sanders read in the file that she was small, as babies often are when born to mothers with Graves' disease, and she was not quite full term.

"Are you happy with her, Ralph?"

"I'm crazy about her, Liz. She's everything a dad could want."

He showed me a black and white picture then. As he handed it to me, I think he guessed he would never get it back. The house in the background was a renovated version of the one I grew up in. Ralph and Irene had taken over the farm when Dad died. The timing was perfect, so Ralph could farm and avoid conscription. The bit of the yard I could see was unrecognizable. The little person in the center of the picture wearing white socks and a fluffy dress looked like a "Marie".

There was a time at the Home when I fell in love with her. My fierce mother protective mode kicked in, and no one, not the director, not God himself, was going to take that baby away from me! But He did, or circumstances did. Whoever it was, the bond wasn't there. I was looking at a photo of Ralph's child, not mine.

"Raise her right, Ralph. She deserves that much."

"I will. I swear."

Talk of the girl brought out the finest side of my brother. He could be a bozo, but I could see the tender father love all over his face. He looked around the room, obviously wanting to end this emotional conversation.

"So, you've done well, Liz. You're making it!"

"I guess I am, whatever "it" is. I'm moving forward. A doctor at the hospital explained it like this. Somewhere, there's a house named "Regret". I can visit there, but I don't have to move in."

"My past is the same. I regret it a lot, but I don't have to think of it all the time. Just so you know, I admire you, Sis. It's been a long road."

Before he left, he handed me a package from Aunt Betty in Penticton. He said it was a keepsake Aunt Flo had insisted they send to me. I placed it on the table. I would open it after my brother left.

He stopped at the door. No tears from me, but his eyes were shiny.

"Proud of you."

I nodded and smiled. I could have left it on that sweet note, but something was resting heavily on my mind.

"Ralph, that day you dropped me off at the Home, I said something awful. I said I could see a lot of our dad in you."

The way he ducked his head let me know he well remembered those biting words.

"I didn't mean it. I was scared, and looking for someone to blame. You're not a bit like him. You never have been."

He stared out through the screen on the door for a moment. I could tell this had been festering for a long while.

"Thanks, Liz, that means a lot."

"Till we meet again," I said, and I watched him from the screen door as he went back around the house to his car.

Marj rushed in as soon as he left. "I was worried. I know this could be the hardest meeting of all for you."

"I'm okay, Marj! In fact, I'm rich!" I held up the envelope of cash.

"I'll take you to the bank on Monday."

"But I'm not putting it all in an account. I'm keeping some of it to buy me a sewing machine of my own!"

The sewing jobs continued to come in, and Marj suggested I would make more money if I quit the coffee shop, and sewed full time. I shook my head. I needed to be with people, and the job Buck offered me was perfect.

I was grateful Buck was working with me on a shift one noon hour when a couple of guys came in. They appeared to be friends and were having a quiet lunch together, but somehow in the middle of their sandwiches and coffee, their hot tempers flared. The smaller man had murder in his eyes, and he stood up so fast, his chair fell over with a bang. The other met the challenge, leaping to his feet, and shaking his fist. Buck was right there, towering over both of them.

"Take it outside, you idiots!"

The smaller man who already had a black eye, probably from carousing the night before, told Buck, "This guy is cruisin' for a bruisin'!" I had not heard that saying before, and it struck me funny. True to form, I burst out laughing, too loud and too long. The skinny, taller man was wearing a beanie, and he hopped around his opponent with his fists circling in the air. "And I got a knuckle sandwich for you!"

Well, I hadn't heard that one either, and I couldn't help it. I hee-hawed like a donkey. As Buck opened the door and kicked them both out, I was doubled over laughing, trying to get control. Buck joined in, whether at me or with me, I don't know. It was so ridiculous, the rest of the customers got into it. It was a hilarious moment, the most fun I've ever had at work. Through the front windows of the shop, we could see the men outside pushing, shoving, and swearing at each other.

Buck yelled out, "Free pie on the house!" I quickly cut the pies in sixes, and Buck served each table. I don't know why, but this was my kind of entertainment. It was more fun than *Abbot and Costello* at the movie theatre on a Saturday afternoon!

AND THEN WE
WERE THREE

G ladys was the outpatient who moved in with Marj and me. Our local Outpatient Program was a growing and glowing success, probably because the patients were handpicked, and designated as most likely to succeed. As time went on, more and more patients were discharged and successfully resumed life in the real world, through the friendship and guidance of hosts like Marj. Unfortunately, not everyone had this level of support. In many cases, patients from around the province were rushed out without a re-entry plan, and necessities were not provided. The results were disastrous and heart-breaking.

I was privileged to be included in our ever-improving Outpatients Program. There was now a fine-tuned preparation procedure in place that was much more sensible than simply walking out one afternoon, as I had done. On that day, I was still wearing the hospital canvas uniform, and we had no idea where I could find employment.

For Gladys, it was different. The program staff arranged for a dry cleaning company in the city to hire her temporarily when she got out. It was on a trial basis, which was fair to all. With that option in place, Gladys was trained for a couple of weeks at the hospital dry cleaners, so she could more confidently take on duties at her job on the outside. Another item on the checklist was assisting Gladys in choosing and ordering some clothing from the catalogue, so that when she walked out, she would not be identified as a patient from the hospital.

The beauty parlor was next. Until that time, Gladys had an unflattering hairstyle. There was no style to it. Her hair was black and poker-straight, cut off squarely just below her ears. The top was swept across her forehead and secured with a bobby pin.

It was decided that curls would be just the thing, and so for the first time ever, Gladys endured the application of a permanent. The transformation was over the top. When the hairdresser held a mirror so Gladys could see herself, she squealed like a little girl, and kept repeating, "Oh my stars! Oh, my stars!"

The perm was done in the morning. After lunch, she dressed in a bright blue dress and new white shoes. The staff gathered around to wish her well.

"Goodbye!"

"Good luck!"

"You're so pretty!"

It was probably the happiest day of Gladys' life. Before we left, the program manager insisted on taking a picture of Marj, Gladys, and me. She had us stand in front of the stone chapel, a perfect backdrop for a send-off. Being the tallest, I stood in the middle with my arm on each of their shoulders, and we were grinning from ear to ear. I was thrilled to be part of this adventure. Gladys was the star of the show, and Marj was beaming like a mother hen.

We were off! Gladys waved from the back seat of Marj's old car to the folks who had gathered in the parking lot. I spied Lily hiding behind the program manager. No one was going to make her into the Outpatient! We stopped for strawberry ice cream at the Chinese café on our way home to celebrate. Marj was making it a tradition.

Gladys was elated to have a room of her own. For me, looking on, it was like reliving my experience the first night on my break for freedom. Marj hung a small mirror on the wall so Gladys could get used to her brand-new look.

The Outpatients Program was expanding, and Marj was the only host so far to have two guests. Our reputation for being steady, thorough workers was the highest recommendation of all to the prospective employers.

According to Marj, the Outpatients Program was well underway, and the officials were thrilled with its success. The activities we had been trying to implement at the hospital were going well.

Patients were gaining work experience, as I had done, by spending time in the different departments of the workforce at the hospital.

About this time, and especially in 1952, a formidable army of volunteers descended on the hospital. They were ladies from various places on the outside who had planned and organized, jumped through the hoops, and were eager to make a difference to the lonely and abandoned patients of the Saskatchewan Hospital.

They had been gathering gift items and dropping them off in the past at Christmas time. Occasionally, a musical group would come through to various wards to offer a lift. But this was different - a force of bustling females with a myriad of talents and ideas. They came by the carload, brought lunches, craft supplies, and held parties and dances. Whatever they had, they gave: cooking classes, games, visiting, book reading, songs, and concerts.

The results were phenomenal. Patients who had not spoken for months or even years, opened up and responded with smiles and a willingness to make eye contact. There were art classes - just some fun painting opportunities - that produced amazing results. The pictures were displayed on the walls. The volunteer program exploded, to the point that the activity department at the hospital also expanded in ways never attempted before.

I noticed Lily was in the center of it all, not taking part in the activities, but explaining hospital trivia to the volunteers. The ladies with whom I had shared a room in the Women's Ward, attended a craft class, all three of them together. They outwardly ignored the volunteers' efforts to include them, but they were present just the same.

The attitudes on the outside were changing. The volunteers spread the word. Patients at the hospital were real people, and were not to be feared, but rather to be valued and encouraged. God bless those volunteers!

As the weeks and months and years went by, the hospital became a different place. There continued to be, of course, very ill patients who were unable to participate, but the general transformation was remarkable. What a change from the grim place it was in the '40s when I landed there at twenty years of age, abandoned, ill, and depressed.

I found myself extra busy as the hospital was buzzing with classes and sessions. I was often asked to come to help on my days off. They encouraged one on one interaction, such as playing cards and other games like crokinole.

I continued my cherished job at Buck's coffee shop, and completed sewing jobs as they came in. I had regained my confidence. Surprisingly, perhaps because of our shaky beginning, Helen and I forged a friendship that extended beyond being employed at the same place. We tried bowling on a Saturday afternoon, and met a couple of other single women who joined us. We went for a pop after, surrounded by teenagers. I had missed that era, as we were in the throes of the Dirty Thirties when I was a teen. We had been in survival mode, with not even two cents for a treat.

I was crazy about western movies after Helen and I went to the rollicking musical, *Calamity Jane*, starring Doris Day. Her romance with Wild Bill Hickok kept us so entertained, I wanted to go again the next weekend. I coaxed Helen to come to *Gunsmoke* on the big screen, the story of a young gunslinger who helped a rancher and his daughter save their land. The shows were harmless, with lots of horses, guns, and shoot 'em up episodes.

Helen said she favored war movies, and had seen one called *Walking My Baby Back Home*. She hoped I would go with her so she could see it a second time, but I refused because I avoided anything to do with the war. I was determined not to let my thoughts turn back to Ray Hutton. It was past time for me to get over those memories, and I would, but I wasn't ready just yet.

Movies were cheap, and Marj encouraged me to go since I enjoyed them so much. She said, "You didn't have any fun for all those years in the hospital, and you have a lot of catching up to do."

I offered to buy her ticket, if she would accompany me to *The Redhead from Wyoming* when it came out. Since Marj was (or had been) a redhead, she saw the fun in attending that particular show. We had a great time ducking smoke and bullets, through to riding with the happy couple into the sunset at the end.

One evening, Marj and I looked at the now well-worn list of goals laid out for the Outpatients Program. We had pretty well covered all the bases, as I had "eased into normal living", to the point that my former hospital days were a distant blur.

Gladys was easing in, too. Marj did an expert job of coaching her, for example, to refrain from eating while she was cooking, and to religiously take her daily medication without fail. Marj was quick to compliment Gladys on her progress, her neat room, and her appearance. Despite lacking confidence, Gladys had a winning way about her. We were as pleased as she was, when she made caring friends through work. She was sweet on a guy at the store next door to the dry cleaners, and told us she went there every day on the pretext of buying lifesavers. She had a purse full of them, but it must have paid off, as he asked her to go to a movie one Friday night. As we got her ready to go, she was nervous and excited at the same time, repeating her old line, "Oh my stars! Oh, my stars!"

She also bought lots of jawbreakers. They were cheap, three for a cent, and we all enjoyed them. They were hard to resist. The tiny coriander seed at the end was the reward. I was as bad as Gladys for buying jawbreakers. Like going to the movies, I was catching up on things I had missed.

The progressive developments at the hospital brought me joy. At the same time as the Outpatients Program became successfully established, antipsychotic drugs were introduced worldwide. This made it possible for numerous patients to be discharged back to their families and home communities. Still more patients from the province were streaming in, possibly to benefit from the advanced drugs being offered, and the ever-present issue of overcrowding increased.

I continued my work and living at Marj's, as well as helping out with the activities at the hospital. I reported for appointments regularly, where my thyroid levels were noted and medication continued. I did not have any particular personal goals, but as the years slipped away, I began to wish for something more. I had been given so much. It was time to give back.

WANTED: A HOUSEKEEPER

I took a little sit down one afternoon while I was cleaning the kitchen. The Family Herald had just arrived in the mail. On a whim, I opened the last page to check out the Classified ads. The Personal column was always good for a laugh, as the desperate offers for marriage were hilarious, and I marked them to read aloud to Marj and Gladys at supper time. Almost as if it was meant to be, my eyes were suddenly riveted on an ad in the Help Wanted section. I read and re-read it, then cut it out with the scissors. I would share this one when the others came home.

"WANTED: Housekeeper for a family of five, children ages three to 14, located on a farm near McKeen, Saskatchewan." The ad refused to leave my mind all day. Could I do it? Would they take me? By the time Marj came home from work, I was pretty well hired, and on my way, at least in my mind.

I tried to be casual about it, "What do you think, Marj?"

"I'm thinking, why not!" We told Gladys, and all three of us sat at the kitchen table with a pen and a writing pad, trying to choose just the right words for my reply.

I wondered if it was too risky to give up my place at Marj's and the job I loved at the coffee shop. I understood if I left, they couldn't hold the spot for me. If it didn't work out, I couldn't expect to be reinstated if I came running back with my tail between my legs.

At Marj's suggestion, I talked it over with Buck. His response was a handwritten letter of recommendation. He included the line, "Liz Parker is the most outstanding employee I have ever had, and I highly recommend her."

We sent his letter and mine in the mail that afternoon to "Mr. Robert Cleaver, Box 22, McKeen, Sask". I thought of little else as I waited for a reply. Marj had suggested that I add her phone number at the end of the letter, in case he wanted to respond that way.

Three days later, the phone rang. I assumed it was for Marj, as Gladys and I seldom received telephone calls. But it was for me, and the voice on the other end of the line was deep and rather unfriendly. He confirmed I was Liz Parker, and said he would like to hire me for the housekeeper job, if I was still interested. I was jumping out of my skin.

I tried to keep my voice down. "You betcha! Yes, for sure!" He sounded businesslike, and much less enthusiastic than I was. He said he would come for me the following Monday, and we made arrangements for him to pick me up at ten o'clock in the morning, in front of Marj's house.

I didn't eat for the rest of the day. I went from room to room and couldn't settle on getting anything done. I had to tell someone, so I phoned Ralph. He had given me his number, back when I became an outpatient. Over the years he kept his distance, probably because of Marie. I had determined never to bother him, but this was something to share.

He was warm on the phone and wished me luck. After that, I settled down and concentrated on doing a little packing. That afternoon I sewed myself a skirt, a peasant blouse and a blue gingham apron.

I had a shift the next day, so I announced my news to Buck when I arrived in the morning. We were busy that noon hour. As the lunch crowd streamed in, a tall man hurriedly entered and sat with his back to the kitchen. He wore a brown fedora, adjusted at a slant that somewhat obscured the side of his face. As he appeared to be in a hurry, I went right over, held my pencil and order pad, and asked my usual question, "Hi, what will it be for you?"

He turned a little more towards the window and said, "I'll have pie and coffee for two. I'm hoping the waitress will join me." Being the only waitress there, I knew he meant me. I hesitated for just a second and then I punched him hard on the shoulder.

"Can't fool your sister, Ralph!" We both laughed as Buck came over to our table and I introduced him to my brother. Buck waved his hand, and pointed to the chair across from Ralph. "Sit down, Goh-jus. Pie and coffee coming right up."

Ralph had come in person to wish me well. We both got a kick out of him trying to fool me. That's the kind of big brother I had always wanted, but the hard times and the distance had changed all that for us. I told him all the details, what the ad said, and the arrangements for me to get to McKeen. He said it was a small town, and he had been there once when he was a teenager.

Buck told me to grab my coat and get out of there. As he smothered me in a big bear hug, he patted my back. "Good luck, Goh-jus!"

Back in my sunroom, I gave Ralph a parcel that contained the Christmas gifts I had made and wrapped to send in the mail. My knitting needles had been clicking for a couple of weeks, long before the job came up. I made double thick mitts for Ralph, with warm, heavy-duty wool. I remembered winters were cold on the farm. I knit a green scarf in a cable design for Irene. It was time I reached out to her, as there was no love lost between us. For Marie...oh yes, for Marie. That took some time and effort, as I wanted it to be the perfect gift. I looked around the stores to see what was out there for young girls. I also checked the catalogue for the latest designs and found exactly what I was looking for. A hat with a pom-pom, and a scarf with a fringe. I made it in white wool, with blue trim exactly like the set pictured in the Wishbook. Marj said the one I made looked nicer.

I asked Ralph if he had told Marie the truth. He appeared relieved to give me a positive answer. "Yes, I did—we both did. She was sitting right there between us, and we told her the whole story."

"And how did she take it?"

My brother will never get the Nobel peace prize for knowing what to say and how to say it.

He looked at his boots, and answered, "Well she cried and cried, and said she wants us to be her real parents. She had heard about adoption from another girl at school. I asked her if she would come and meet you."

"And..."

She said, "No! Never! I won't. She ruined my life!"

I didn't speak my thoughts out loud, but I was thinking, "Dear brother Ralph, don't you know that cut my heart like a knife? You could have spared me her exact words."

He looked up at the v-joint ceiling and said helplessly, "She's just a kid, Liz, she'll come around."

I managed to say, "Well she's got some spark in her, doesn't she, Ralph? I wonder where she gets that from!"

He left soon after that. I wondered what Marie would think of her Christmas gift from the one who ruined her life. Before he said goodbye, he asked if I had everything I needed for my venture. I had ordered overshoes from the catalogue, as well as a warm winter coat, which would be sent to Cleavers' address. I assured him I was set.

I sat in my armchair looking out at the bare trees. We had raked up the leaves a couple of weeks ago. In the mornings, you could feel winter on its way. The snow would fly soon, but by then I would be on the Cleaver farm, hopefully adding warmth in more ways than one.

As I sat alone, I pondered Marie's words, those four painful words, "She ruined my life." Oh, little one. Tell me who ruined whose life! If there had been no baby, there well may not have been Graves' disease, or the years in the hospital. I canceled that thought before it was completely formed, because I have never, and will never, blame that innocent baby for my undoing.

Gladys usually went to bed early. I told Marj over a cup of tea what Marie had said. Her comment surprised me, "Someone said those exact words to me one time."

"A boyfriend?"

"No, a husband."

When you know someone all your life, you know that person's history. But when you meet later on, as Marj and I did, we know only what we choose to share. I assumed Marj had always been single. She went on to tell me she was "divorced", a status not popular in our society. Only a few people were aware of it, as her marriage broke up long ago. She met her husband's secret girlfriend by chance, and when confronted, he accused Marj of ruining his life.

Marj said with a grin, "Once we found out about each other, the other woman and I left him in the dust. Right after that, I got the job at the hospital, and saw so many worse off than I was. It helped me with perspective and to get back my confidence. Look at me now!"

Hearing about her experience helped me bear Ralph's report of what Marie thought of me. I looked ahead to unfolding possibilities. There was a family of kids needing love and support. I hoped I was up for the task. I would give it my best shot. Marj promised to stand behind me all the way, as I embarked on this new adventure.

I watched Monday morning dawn bright and clear, as the sun rose on a beautiful fall day. It was after seven, but I had been awake for ages. To pass the time, I scrubbed the kitchen within an inch of its life, and then moved through each room. Marj would have a sparkling house to remember me by! Gladys and Marj made me promise to write and let them know how I liked living on a farm. They left for work, and I feverishly continued my cleaning spree. Marj gave me a suitcase, in which I carefully packed my clothes, aprons, knitting needles, and wool. She threw in a couple of recipe books.

"You never know what they'll have there, Liz, and these recipes are tried and true."

We placed my sewing machine in a corner of the living room, and covered it with a pineapple pattern crocheted table cloth. She promised it would be safe and untouched till I claimed it again.

At 9:30 I couldn't stand to stay inside any longer, so I waited outside, eagerly watching for the farm truck. He was right on time, and the truck made a gurgling sound as it came to a stop. I hurried out to the street from my perch on the step, put my suitcase on the ground, and extended my hand.

"Hi, I'm Liz. Liz Parker."

He put my suitcase in the truck box, and away we went. The truck seemed to be suffering a little. The dour look on Robert Cleaver's face made me hope it was the truck, and not me that was causing that dark look. He wasn't much of a talker.

When I thought we were heading out of the city, he turned down a side street, and stopped in front of a shabby building with the sign, "Bob's Transmissions." Just like a man not to say why we were stopping. He could have said, "As you can tell, the truck needs some help. I'm picking up a few parts that it's going to need." Instead, he simply slammed the driver's door and disappeared inside the shop. I sat there imagining what he could have said, and in about twenty minutes he came back carrying a heavy-looking truck part that he put in the back beside my suitcase.

We started again with a cough and a sputter of the engine. I was glad I'd worn my work shoes. If we ended up hoofing it, I would be okay. I waited till we were on the outskirts of town before I said anything.

"Mr. Cleaver, I'm excited about meeting your kids."

He nodded, but said not a word. I tried again. "I appreciate you giving me the job," He looked straight ahead, both hands on the wheel as he kept the old crate moving down the center of the gravel road.

Silence is just not my thing. "So, I'll tell you a little about myself. I'm 32 years old and spent the early years of my childhood in Belle Valley, south of Stillwater."

He glanced over at me, and I took that as permission to keep talking. "I was raised by an aunt." I didn't want to divulge any details about my dad, the abuse, or the alcohol. I didn't want him to think I was from bad stock.

I continued, "She tried to raise me right, to be truthful and honest. I can promise you I will do my best in that way with your kids."

I guess he finally decided to loosen up a bit, "That's what I want. And don't be easy on them. They don't need to be served. They've learned how to pitch in and work. That's what I expect."

"Good for you," I said, "I agree." I went on to say I believed in a clean and organized house. "I like to cook and bake, as I told you in my letter, and meals will be on time. You say when."

I wish I could say I sat quietly with my hands folded, watching the scenery for the rest of the trip. I couldn't stand the awkward atmosphere, so I chattered on about my work at the coffee shop, and I even mentioned going to *Gunsmoke* on the weekend. I carefully avoided any mention of the Saskatchewan hospital. I figured that was a sure-fire way to get fired before I even got to the job!

We drove through McKeen about noon, and he asked if I wanted to stop for lunch. As I had brought along a fair bit of cash, I said, "Sure. I'm buying."

He looked at me strangely and raised his eyebrows as if to say, "Are you sure?"

He angle-parked in front of a café that had an OPEN sign in the window. Special of the day was fried chicken and biscuits. The coffee was welcome, not as good as the smooth java Buck's machine put out, but I was ready for a jolt after being awake half the night.

The food arrived at our table quickly, and we didn't waste any time eating. I stacked the dishes as any well-trained waitress would, and left the money and a small tip. Back in the truck, he had the good sense to say thanks. I was thinking if he didn't, how on earth could I expect to teach manners to the kids?

He asked if I needed anything from town, and I told him I had picked up anything I thought I'd need back in the city. He volunteered that he had stocked up the kitchen with groceries on the weekend. I was happy to hear that. "Have groceries, will cook!"

I caught him looking over at me a couple of times as we traveled. Probably checking out my eyes. I decided it was none of his business. Some things are personal, and it appeared to me he was carrying a lot of secrets. I would, too.

The farm was only five miles from town. He politely carried my suitcase into the house, and told me I would be sharing a room upstairs with his girl. I couldn't help asking about her, as Marie had been on my mind for the last two days since I had seen Ralph.

"Oh, you have a girl? How old is she?"

"She's ten. She knows how to work!"

"And the others?"

"All boys."

It was a conversation we should have had in the truck as we rolled along, but he was not one to leak any information. I guessed I would find out about them for myself.

I heard the truck leave the yard, and in about ten minutes or less, it roared back into the lane. Mr. Cleaver and a pudgy little boy of about three or four appeared in the doorway.

"Here's Mac."

I went down on my knees. "Hi, Mac. I'm Liz."

He wasn't the least bit shy, but he didn't say a word as he followed me inside. It wasn't long till I had checked out the cupboards, and Mac was standing on a chair by the table stirring cookie dough. I was wearing one of my new aprons, and somehow felt like I belonged in that kitchen.

The house and the whole situation were better than I had hoped. It was a humble home, but I wasn't looking for fancy. I had always lived in a clean but simple home with make-do furniture.

Time was flying, and I expected the kids after three. I wondered how they got to school, and where it was. I swept the floor and tidied the place. Mac took me for a walk around the yard, where I saw a few cats and met Skipper the dog. Mac was my silent partner. I figured he had been spending too much time with that dad of his. Neither one of them knew how to carry on a conversation.

I got the fire started in the cookstove and filled the kettle. I made myself a cup of tea, and poured a little in a cup for Mac, topped up with plenty of milk and sugar. I showed him how to stir it and as we both stirred our tea, I said, "Mac, say thanks."

He did. He said it clear as day. "Thanks!" Okay, there was nothing wrong with his speech, he just needed practice.

We got the cookies in the oven about the time we heard children's voices in the yard. I ran out to the step and stood there, watching a horse and buggy coming down the lane. I loved them as soon as I saw them. I can't explain it. I was a woman on a mission, and I was in the right place at the right time.

I fell for the girl, as I knew I would. Her name was Dot. She was tough, watching me carefully, and I had no doubt she could set me straight if she thought I was out of line. By evening though, I could already see she was a hurting little girl, lonely and needing a mother's love. The older two boys were friendly and Nick, the closest in age to Mac, was a fetching little guy with freckles and a missing front tooth.

They set to work at their afterschool chores, without argument or complaint. The fact that the kids were respectful and well trained proved to me they had been raised by decent parents. I wondered about their mother, and how long she had been gone. The information would come out sooner than later. It always does with kids.

I was in my glory as the week passed. Making meals, preparing school lunches, organizing their clothes, making sure the kids were clean and their teeth brushed before bed, tidying up at the end of the day. I knew how to wash a separator. I had helped with that job countless times at the Rogers' house, and I used scalding water to rinse the milk pails, before hanging them in the porch for the morning.

Mr. Cleaver slept in the living room, as Dot and I shared one of the two bedrooms upstairs, the one he would have normally had. So, I made sure I went upstairs fairly early after the work was done.

The following Monday, my boss asked if I wanted to go to town for groceries. I said, "Sure," grabbed my purse, and hopped in the truck in less than a minute. I had a letter with a stamp on it, ready to drop in the post office to Marj and Gladys. They would be dying to know how things were going.

As we drove out the lane with Mac plopped between us, I got right to it. "Mr. Cleaver, I've been here a week, and I need to know if you are pleased with my work."

He nodded.

"If there's anything I'm doing wrong, or anything you disagree with, please tell me now."

He almost smiled.

"Well, don't call me Mr. Cleaver. I can't stand it."

"Okay. Robert."

He nodded. It was so annoying that he wouldn't talk. It didn't take me long to think back to my silent days. When I was admitted to the hospital, I was grieving. Grieving the loss of my baby, my appearance, my freedom, my aunt - all of those things - along with hormones gone crazy from the thyroid issue. The circumstances had silenced me, and the pressure of the pent-up unspoken pain was almost more than I could bear. I realized Robert was grieving, too. I would have mercy.

I chatted with Mac and moved him to my knee, so he could see out as we drove along. There were some horses in the field outside of town. He got all excited and said, "Gid-up, gid-up!" This little lad loved horses, and I tucked away that bit of information. Planted in my brain was an idea for a bedtime story for the little boys.

The farm was the place for me! Aunt Flo's house had been on the edge of town, and I spent endless happy days with the Rogers kids running around the countryside, building a playhouse in the bushes, and cooking food outside.

Mac and I took to going for walks in the pasture, as the fall days were still warm enough for afternoon hikes. I pulled him on a Radio Flyer wagon at the beginning of our forays, and then he got out and walked along beside me. That way we could go further, he didn't get too tired and we met up with the wagon on the way home.

There was an intriguing junk pile in the yard that spoke of days gone by. There was an old stove, discarded when a better one replaced it, and a table made of solid wood with a deep crack down the middle. Refinished and repaired, that table could be a beauty.

I loved the freedom that I sensed in body and soul. I felt like a different person than the one who spent eight years in the hospital. Like a cat, I maybe had nine lives. The first one was on the farm where I was born, second, with Aunt Flo, third, the dreadful series of events at the Home and the hospital, fourth, an outpatient with Marj, and now fifth, housekeeper and substitute mom. Oh heck, that's only five lives used up, still four to go!

An old car was retired deep in the bush south of the house. Mac and I climbed into it, and I let him drive. He planted his feet on the bare springs of the driver's seat, and vigorously spun the wheel from side to side while I cheered him on, "Go faster, Mac! You can do it!"

He loved driving so much that he took Nick out there the next Saturday morning. When I looked out the window, they were just a-rattling down their imaginary road in the old car that didn't have a wheel left on it.

When I'm happy, I sing. I discovered Mac was an eager little singer, and so we sang as we walked in the pasture and when we worked in the kitchen. I taught him the words, and I loved hearing him sing along. He took to the song, "Billy Boy", and sang it for the kids when they got home from school.

Can she bake a cherry pie, Billy Boy, Billy Boy?
Can she bake a cherry pie, charming Billy?
She can bake a cherry pie,
Quick as a cat can wink an eye,
She's a young thing and cannot leave her mother.

The kids nearly died laughing when Mac managed to wink as he sang about the cat. He was such a great little entertainer that his siblings, even the two older boys, went into gales of giggles. That's how it is supposed to be in a family.

I was trying to inject fun into life at the Cleavers. It wasn't hard to do. I was happy, and my cup was full. Dot fell in love with the song, "In the Blue Canadian Rockies". Their teacher had described the Rocky Mountains during social studies and the song fit in perfectly. I wrote the words for her in a notebook, and we often sang it, as it was a pretty tune and she had a dream of seeing those mountains.

Oh, what is it about music that changes the mood of a day and takes us places we can never go? I had depended on music throughout my life to carry me through. It was satisfying to foster a love for music in these children.

The cold weather came, as we knew it would. We made sure the kids had warm winter wear. My knitting needles were busy, and I had almost used up the ample supply of wool Marj had tucked in the suitcase at the last minute.

Nick's birthday was a special celebration. He helped bake his chocolate birthday cake, with a little money hidden in some of the pieces.

I had been a storyteller since I helped take care of the younger Rogers children. I loved spinning a tale, and holding them captive as the story unfolded. I was certain Mac and Nick would go for cowboy stories, so I started with a version of my favorite movie, *Calamity Jane*. I set up Wild Bill Hickok to be their hero, and there was nothing that cowboy couldn't do! He was wild and tough, and he used his gun only to protect innocent people and cattle.

He once saved a little boy from dangerous bank robbers, just in the nick of time. All credit for that spectacular rescue was due to Buckshot, the fastest horse in Texas. You couldn't even see his hooves when he ran.

Another story included two brothers named Lucky and Tex, and I threw in a dog that looked exactly like Skipper. It was Calamity Jane who finally found them, lost and alone. Sure enough, Wild Bill galloped into the canyon in a cloud of dust where he killed a rattler poised to strike. Believe it or not, the dog rode home on Calamity Jane's horse, sitting on his haunches behind the saddle!

There was a proper moral to each Old West story. Before bed, the boys begged for "Wild Bill". If I left them with a cliff hanger, they couldn't stand it.

"Please just finish it, so we can get to sleep," Nicky begged. I noticed the older kids were listening to the stories, too, so I spiced them up with a little romance or humor that flew over the little boys' heads.

I figured things were going well for me at my new job. I wished Robert would give some affirmation, but he was still in his dark funk much of the time. Staring at nothing. I had seen that look too often at the hospital, and with the kids' help, I kept the house lively in the evenings, yet not overly noisy. I had a feeling Robert Cleaver just needed time, as I had when my world fell apart.

I taught Dot to embroider and to knit. I felt like I was reliving my childhood, but this time I was Aunt Flo, and Dot was me. She caught on quickly to whatever I taught her, including cooking and baking. She insisted on writing down recipes so she could always have them. I quickly observed that she was an amiable kid at the core, and she tried hard to please me. We each carried an empty spot in our hearts. I knew she wasn't Marie, and she knew I wasn't her mom, but we were substitutes, and our bond held firm.

When Dot was away at school, I created a hat with pom-poms and a scarf with a fringe, using the leftover white and blue wool. It was identical to the one I had made for Marie, and Dot was elated. She was struggling to be accepted at school, and she thought if she wore the right clothes, the girls would treat her better. I wondered how Marie got along at school, and if Irene was a loving mom to her.

Oh, what a cold winter it was! Saskatchewan's memorable storm of '55 kept us fighting the elements for three days. The blizzard finally blew itself out on the third day, and snowplows roared into the yard. I took Nick and Mac out on the step to watch. There was a whole cavalcade of big tractors with V-ploughs on the front. They had a system where one machine closely followed another, taking great bites out of the heavy snowdrifts in the yard.

Suddenly, I heard an unintelligible sound coming out of Mac as Nicky yelled, "Liz, Mac is stuck to the railing!" And he was - stuck by the tongue!

Oh, my precious boy. You are not the first or the last little prairie chicken who has frozen his tongue to a steel post! I darted into the house, grabbed a cup of water from the water pail, and poured it on his tongue. It immediately let go, but there was blood in his mouth and he sobbed in my arms as I carried him inside the house. Nick remained on the step watching the machines with little boy fascination.

Mac got special treatment for the rest of the day. I told him a wound in your mouth is very painful, but it heals quickly. A couple of cowboy stories hastened the recovery.

One afternoon, the kids raced into the house, reporting that the Bells had a frightening experience on the way to school. They had a light cutter and fast horses, and somehow the runners on the right side went up on a bank of snow that was a little too steep. The cutter completely tipped over, and Louise told them it was really scary. Coals from the little stove had spilled out, and Louise's young brother, Archie, had a burn on his leg. Their dad had to lift his kids through the door, which was facing the sky. Stan then managed to push himself up and out, and the three of them were able to shove the cutter right side up again. The well-trained team knew enough to stop when it happened, or it could have been a lot worse.

That night before bed, Nicky, who tried never to show weakness in front of his older brothers, asked if it might happen to them some time on their way to school. I told him it wasn't likely, as our cutter was heavier and our team, Danny and Moe, were careful. I also assured him if it did happen, his dad would safely rescue them just as Stan Bell had done for his kids.

There was a large box of used clothes stored in the closet of the bedroom I shared with Dot. I went through it one day when Mac was taking a nap and the older kids were at school. I discovered just what I was looking for, but I needed to ask Robert's permission to repurpose them. He hesitated when I asked, but looked at the floor and said, "Use anything you want." At the bottom of the box were some dresses, which I dared not touch.

It didn't take long to iron some plaid shirts, and assess what fabric I could salvage from them. I created a paper pattern from shirts that currently fit Nick and Mac. I had in my mind two little cowboys dressed in shirts and fringed vests. The boys beamed when they tried on their western duds.

Then there was the Christmas concert. I loved every minute of it, all the work and the preparation. I made sure the kids memorized their parts for the plays and learned the words of the songs, and I was determined they would look their best. I sewed a white shirt for Roy, and he was handsome as a prince. He and I built a rapport, as I could see he and his dad were on the verge of tangling almost all the time. His hair was long and unruly, but I coaxed him to let me trim it before the concert. He was pleased with the result. Thanks to my experience at the hospital beauty parlor, I could cut hair like a pro.

I taught Will how to use the sewing machine. He had a real knack for it, and I told him some of the most outstanding sewers in the world were men. Some were shoemakers, harness makers, and tailors of complicated projects like sewing men's suits and formal wear.

The older boys had an addiction to playing crib, once I taught them how. I shared my old deck of Eifel Tower cards and the cribbage board that Ewald and I had made in the workshop. That was another world, another planet, and another life. I believe I had designated that era as the third of my cat lives. I looked over my shoulder at the past, and I had to admit those years at the hospital were not wasted. I had learned some life skills and some important life lessons in that place.

Every once in a while, my mood took a dive. I had no explanation for it, as I had never before experienced such fulfillment and day to day happiness as I did while working as a housekeeper for that family. I sometimes had a down day and then managed to pop right back up, better than ever. Hormones are fickle. They take you up and down on a roller coaster - high, low, dip, up again and around.

In November, I had a fleeting urge to somehow get a ride into Marj's and get a checkup at the hospital. I should have done so before I left for the job, but it came up so suddenly, and I was so excited that it never crossed my mind. Just when I decided I needed to get to Dr. Sanders, life got so very busy on the farm. Winter came, the storm, birthday celebrations, the Christmas concert, and Christmas itself. We were flying high, all of us, except Robert, I guess. The first Christmas without his wife was borne in his usual silence.

The kids and I made it a Christmas to remember. We loaded the table with yummy food, and we played games and shared gifts. With encouragement, Will and Dot made stick horses for Nick and Mac. They stuffed socks to make the horses' heads, added ears and eyes, and yarn for manes, and then hid them behind the tree for a Christmas morning surprise. Robert ordered cowboy hats from the catalogue, and what a sight Tex and Lucky were on Christmas Day, as they rode those horses upstairs and down!

Just after New Year's, I crashed. I had shaken off the telltale symptoms that I briefly remembered from 1943. When I finally acknowledged the problem to myself, I planned to phone Marj to come and get me. I didn't get that done, and I simply did not know how to march up to Robert and say, "Please Mr. Cleaver, would you kindly drop me off at the mental hospital?"

I hoped it would wear off, that I could get a grip, and then...I don't know exactly. I guess it was the mania, as they called it when I lost my sanity back at the Home for Unwed Mothers. I left a note for

Dot in our room, that much I remembered. I felt guilt and despair for letting down the kids I had grown to love so much. I wondered what Robert Cleaver must have thought of me. And what would happen to the kids now? That was a dark time for me. My entire life had been made up of repeating eras of dark and light, with nothing in between.

FULL CIRCLE

I opened my eyes to see a high white ceiling above me. Again. Dr. Sanders, strong and steady, took my hand in his. "Liz, you're safe and you're going to be okay." This time I knew exactly where I was. No shock, no questions. I had come full circle. I landed here the first time and worked my way out. Now I was back. After all these years, I was once again confined within the familiar and formidable walls of the hospital.

I turned to look at the doctor who had seen me through so many years of my journey. He looked older and his voice was compassionate. I felt a sadness come over me that I had not felt for a long while.

"I'll never get out again, will I." It was a statement, not a question.

"Oh, Liz, of course, you will! You've been doing so well. We know what happened, and it wasn't your fault. We didn't keep a close enough eye on those thyroid levels. They topped out again, and you had an episode. We can get you back on track faster than you think."

He had never lied to me before. He may have tried to sugar-coat some of his words, but he hadn't lied. He was offering me hope on a silver platter, but I was dousing it with doubt.

"It was great you took that job out at McKeen. Marj has told us how excellent it was for you and for them. She feels guilty that she didn't make sure you came in for tests before you left. You never know with Graves'. Sometimes we never see it again, and sometimes it pops up without much warning."

With his encouraging words, I was able to buck off some of the shame that rode me. I didn't remember everything that happened when I left Cleaver's farm, but I knew it had ended badly. I had burst into the lives of five motherless children to give hope, and then quickly disappeared in disgrace. What that did to them, I couldn't imagine. One day I would meet them again to plead my case, so they would know I didn't abandon them on purpose.

Dr. Sanders assured me that kids are resilient. "They will keep their fond memories of the three or so months you had together and let the rest go." I had to believe him. I knew I had to let it go, too. If I didn't, the crushing weight of my guilt would hinder my healing.

I spent two weeks in the medical ward, where I saw Dr. Sanders each morning. He was right - this was a quicker turnaround. I expected to be put back in the Women's Ward any time, and set to work. How I wished I could go back to my sunroom at Marj's, enjoying my job at the coffee shop and the seamstress work that came my way. I knew when I applied for the housekeeper job that I was risking the loss of my satisfying life, and the opportunities at Marj's. I still couldn't say I was sorry I tried it. My life as an outpatient was almost perfect, but my real run at freedom was the housekeeper job that lasted less than four months.

Marj dropped in to see me one day, and we had a cozy visit. She was, of course, still working at the hospital and now had two female outpatients living with her. Gladys had taken up residence in my sunroom, and Marj assured me my sewing machine was still waiting for me when I got out. Long ago, I had wished Marj could be a friend, and she had become exactly that, supporting me through thick and thin.

One morning when Dr. Sanders came in, he was giddy as a girl. "I've just come up with the best idea I've had in my life. I've found a room for you."

I knew the wards were crowded but had it been that hard to find one bed?

"Not only a room, but the perfect roommate. I think it's a match!"

He went on to describe a female patient, severely debilitated with rheumatoid arthritis, who required a substantial amount of physical care. She had been placed in a single room, near the nurses' desk on Ward 3C.

"When her mother died in 1950, she came here to us, as there was no alternate facility for her long-term care. She's the most uncomplaining soul in this entire hospital, even though she suffers pain all the time. My big concern is that she is depressed and lonely. I can only imagine what a wonderful personality like yours could do to bring her out of herself and give her a renewed love for life."

The reason I applied for the housekeeper job for the Cleaver family was that I wanted to make those motherless children laugh again. Looking back, there had been lots of fun and laughter in my short time with them. I was eager to meet the woman.

Dr. Sanders asked if I wanted to think about it. I shook my head. "What are we waiting for?"

As we walked the lengthy distance to 3C, Dr. Sanders was practically rubbing his hands together with glee. He made the introductions and quickly left us to get acquainted on our own.

At first sight, Wilma looked like a body without a face. Her rheumatoid arthritis had progressed to the point that her shoulders hunched forward, and her head was resting on her chest. The top of her graying hair was what I saw initially. Her arms were stiff at her sides, and her hands deformed. I quickly lowered myself beside her so I could look up into her face.

"Hi, I'm Liz. I'm looking for a friend."

Her voice was weak, but I saw her ready smile and heard her say, "Me, too!"

The room was very small. There was space only for a bed along each wall. Her armchair from her home was situated near the window. She had a small dresser. Perhaps we could share it.

In the beginning, the nurses stopped in often to see to Wilma's needs. Usually, though, I had already made her comfortable in some way, helped her lie down or get up into her armchair so she didn't have to wait. After two or three weeks, I helped Wilma with most of her care, which greatly eased the workload of the staff.

As we got to know each other, our spirits were lifted. Wilma had a very quiet voice, so I had to strain to hear her words. As her head was bent so far forward, the volume she could muster was lost in the folds of her dress. We managed to communicate, to rediscover the lighter side of life, and to laugh. I had been cursed (or blessed) with a loud belly laugh from my childhood. It was my trademark back in my school days and even yet, I wasn't very successful in trying to tone down the volume. One day, Mrs. Davis came hustling in from the nurses' desk not far from our door.

"There's far too much laughing in here!" We knew by her smile she was kidding.

"If I talk too much, Wilma, give me a hand signal to shut up." I could barely see her smile from her folded position. She attempted to point to the window, and I realized she wanted to see out. I was pretty sure I could help her stand, mainly because her condition had made her shorter than she once was, and also, she was light as a feather. When I realized she had no balance at all, I knew I had to pay attention as I supported her with my arm around her back.

It was the river scene again, my favorite view. I told her we could watch the sun set in the evenings over the water. The cars in the distance appeared to be tiny toys as they climbed the hill to the bridge. Closer to our room, we could see the flowered paved pathway and a clear view of the chapel, an exquisite work of art in stone. Every day after that, I helped her stand to look outside. This was her window to the world.

When Dr. Sanders asked us how things were working out, we expressed our thanks. Wilma's friendship meant the world to me, and helping her gave purpose to my day. The doctor's brilliant idea of having us share a room was of benefit to us both, just as he had hoped. Wilma said ours was a match made by Dr. Sanders and the angels.

She preferred that I feed her, as the nurses were always in a rush. Her hands were so bent and twisted that she could no longer hold a spoon. She was a slow eater, and so we took our time and some of our best conversations occurred at mealtime.

A LONG, TALL TEXAN

The first Sunday after I moved in with Wilma, her brother Jarvis appeared for his regular visit. I had been told he was coming, but I wasn't expecting such a good-looking man. I couldn't help but exclaim, "So Wilma, who's this long, tall Texan!"

I extended my hand as I always did when meeting someone. "Hi, I'm Liz. Liz Parker." He was the farmer type, wearing jeans and a plaid shirt with the sleeves rolled up to his elbows. He wore gold-rimmed glasses, and when he smiled, his eyes crinkled up on the sides. His face was tanned from working outside, his hair was dark brown with some grey in his sideburns.

I knew I should make myself scarce, so Wilma could have her anticipated visit with her brother. The timing was perfect, as it was almost time for the two o'clock church service, which I usually attended.

"I shall return later," I told them both, and turned to go out the door. For once, Wilma managed some volume in her voice. "Stop! You're not going anywhere."

I suggested we hunt down a wheelchair, so we could take Wilma outside. She had been cooped up way too long.

Besides the gift of Wilma's friendship, another plus for me was that I got to meet her teenage friend, Linda. She lived on the farm closest to Jarvis and came with him on some Sunday afternoons to brighten Wilma's day. She was a talkative girl, in Grade 11, above average height and well-proportioned. She was always talking about new clothes, hairstyles, homework, and boys, and how much she hated school. We knew that wasn't true, as she talked so much about it. Linda was a breath of fresh air, bringing that outside world inside to us.

The girl had an eye for fashion. She wore bobby socks and kept her saddle shoes polished bright and white. She often played with the plastic-colored pop-beads around her neck, re-forming them to make a long necklace or two short ones. Usually, she popped a few of them together to make a matching pony tail circle.

Our school days were long gone, and Linda refreshed our memories. She loved to hear about our experiences at school, too, especially the boys we liked. Wilma admitted in front of Jarvis, that if she hadn't got sick, she would have chased down a guy who was the hired man at the farm for a while. Linda tried to coax out of me my past romantic history. I didn't share much. The specter of the Home for Unwed Mothers never went away.

I was allowed to make afternoon tea for Wilma and me, heating water on a hot plate near the back of the reception office. One day, I noticed a truck pull up in front of the office door, and a man and a woman came inside. They were farm folks and the man spoke politely.

"We're here to check on a patient."

The nurses were always careful about confidentiality. Mrs. Davis asked, "The patient's name, please?"

"Well, we don't know her name," the man answered, "but it's the old lady who wandered to our farm out near Midling last week."

Mrs. Davis was all ears. "Oh, you're the ones!"

The man asked, "Is she doing okay?"

"Oh yes, she's just fine. She slept for three days when she got back here, but I saw her after breakfast this morning and she was gathering the dishes as she likes to do. So, tell me what happened. Did she just stroll into your yard and knock on the door?"

They both nodded, and the wife said, "She looked exhausted. Her dress had mud on it, and she had bits of grass and leaves in her hair. I thought she must have slept in a ditch."

Mrs. Davis was very interested. "Likely that's true. She was probably trying to get to her old home, but couldn't find the way."

"She asked me how my garden was this year, so I figured she was probably from a farm."

"You're right. She was a hardworking farm woman. Unfortunately, she needs to be here with us, but she does long for home."

"She was famished, and after she ate, I asked if she wanted to lie down and rest."

The husband added, "When I came in the house she was snoring on the couch. We figured she must be from up here. I made the call from my neighbor's phone so as not to upset her."

The wife added, "When the police officer came, she was so agreeable. He said, 'I'll give you a nice ride in my car.' And she hopped in."

Mrs. Davis was enjoying the news. "You folks have been kind, and thank you for coming in to follow up."

She watched them leave the parking lot and said out loud, "Wasn't that nice of them!"

That's when she noticed me. I was feeling awkward as if I shouldn't have been listening in. After all, I was not staff, I was a patient. I picked up the tray to take to our room when Mrs. Davis asked, "Liz, did you know Alice Mallard took a walk last week, all the way to Midling?"

I nodded. The staff was unaware there was a robust grapevine among the patients. We often knew things the nurses never found out about. Of course, we knew of Alice's adventure! All I said was, "I'm so glad she was okay."

One of the most informative messengers on the grapevine was Lily. I wasn't surprised when she popped up near the nurses' desk. There were fewer locked doors now at the hospital, and Lily seemed to be anywhere and everywhere.

"So, you're the Inpatient now like me."

I nodded. "Rub it in, Lily", is what I was thinking.

"Don't worry, the Big Boss says you can be the Outpatient again after Christmas." I hoped her information was accurate, but I was not desperate to leave. I enjoyed my days with Wilma, and helping her made me feel fulfilled as I had at Cleavers.

I had been wondering about Illa and Mrs. Dodds, so I asked Lily how they were doing. Her eyes clouded over. "They're both gone. Gone forever." She quickly turned around and hurried away. As she went, I heard her mumbling, "Gone forever and ever. Amen."

Later in the afternoon, she approached me again.

"I picked a big bunch of flowers today for the chapel."

"Oh, did you put them in water?"

"No, I just laid them in a pile on the bench. I gave them to God."

"Good for you, Lily."

SAFE AND SECURE

Every Sunday afternoon at two o'clock, a short church service was held in the gathering room. Not many attended, maybe ten or fifteen, but I found it a pleasant diversion and it set the day apart from the rest of the week. Ministers from different churches took a turn on a rotation of about four or five weeks.

I kept track of the schedule and took a liking to a young preacher who was always accompanied by his very timid wife. If he had tried to present the dignified minister look, he couldn't have pulled it off, as he had what I can only describe as a round, baby face and a wayward rooster tail that pointed straight up towards heaven. They dressed up for the service, he in a suit, shirt, and tie, no doubt the clothes he had worn to the morning service at his church. She wore a skirt and suit jacket with white wedge sandals.

What I liked most was his sincerity, his excellent singing voice, and his guitar. I found out his name was Ken and hers was Twyla. I often went in a little early and set up the chairs in a semi-circle, and when they brought the box of hymnbooks, I spread them out on the chairs.

As I sang "Leaning on the Everlasting Arms" with the small group of people in the gathering room, I was transported back to Saturday nights in the Thirties when I was a teenager. Aunt Flo usually sent me downtown to deliver whatever jars of milk we had for sale. We didn't bother with a separator. We offered whole milk, and it was a blessing both ways. Our customers needed it for their littlest children, and we certainly could use every penny that came our way. We bought feed for our cow wherever we could get it—whatever we could beg, borrow, or steal to keep her well-conditioned enough to continue producing milk.

On those Saturday evenings, at about eight o'clock, the street meeting people came from another town, and set up on the corner by the Post Office, where the most people were coming and going. The "band" consisted of a woman sitting on a folding chair playing a red and white accordion, and a guitar player. The accordion looked like it was too big for her, but she had a smile on her face and she really could wield that thing around on a fast song. A man strummed a guitar and appeared to be following her lead, tapping his toe in time to the music. He had a leather strap around his neck to hold the guitar in place. The third person was the preacher. I heard him preach before from that same spot, and he was usually clapping his hands to the music, I suppose to keep things rolling.

They sang gospel hymns that I liked, and I remember one night in particular. As I approached, the song they were singing was "Leaning on the Everlasting Arms". That's when I saw Ronnie Galley making fun of them, and yelling as he and his friends passed by. He was leaning to the side, almost falling over, and he leaned further every time they sang the word. He was trying to laugh louder than the music, I expect to distract the few interested folks who were clustered in a small group, singing along. He was what we would call a "heckler", in a political meeting.

I knew Ronnie well from school. He was about 16 at that time, the same as I was. He was tall and skinny as a beanpole, and was known for acting up. I have never hesitated to speak my mind, and it took only four or five long steps for me to catch up to him. He was still clowning around.

"Ronnie Galley, you're making a fool of yourself!"

He stopped laughing long enough to catch his breath and yell out, "Oh, praise the Lord!"

That was enough for me. I lowered my voice but he heard me loud and clear. "Ronnie, there are people here who need this, people who..." At that moment, I noticed the Wilson family in the small crowd that had gathered, standing close to the musicians. Mrs. Wilson was openly crying. I knew they had lost one of their children during that past week, as Aunt Flo had sent me over with fresh bread and a jar of milk. I had Ronnie's full attention as I finished my sentence. "People who have lost everything. They're broken and they are suffering. Don't blame them for trying to find help."

The grin faded from Ronnie's face. I'd had my say, and as I kept walking straight ahead on the sidewalk, I soon realized the boys were walking beside me. My heart softened towards them.

"Things are tough for all of us and even worse for some." No doubt Ronnie had seen the folks back there, including the Wilsons and their skinny kids. I found my milk customers near the store, and it was Ronnie who asked if I wanted to go back with him to join the street meeting.

I was feeling pretty satisfied that I had helped him see the light, and I was amazed that he had such a complete change of heart.

I said, "Sure, let's go!" I told him I could only stop for a little while, because my Aunt Flo had been having spells with her heart and I needed to check on her. Sometimes the street meetings went on quite long, and I wouldn't be staying to the end.

I didn't admit it to Ronnie or to anyone else, but I was looking for help, too. Every day, I worried about my aunt, and every night when I said my prayers, I prayed her heart would hold out. I was not raised to go to church. I didn't know if anyone was listening, but it was worth the chance.

I forced myself out of my daydream of those old Dirty Thirties days, and tuned back into the present. They were singing the last verse, and it sounded better than usual. The minister and his wife had brought several people with them this time, no doubt to beef up the singing, and to visit with us a little when it was over. I joined in, as the hymnbook was still open on my lap.

Oh how sweet to walk in this pilgrim way,
Leaning on the everlasting arms,
Oh how bright the path grows from day to day,
Leaning on the everlasting arms

The music kept taking me back to the street meeting, where I stood beside the chastened Ronnie Galley.

"Leaning, leaning, safe and secure from all alarms." Since moving in with Wilma, my life was better. My fears of mentally losing it all again were slowly subsiding. Her peaceful nature was rubbing off on me. I felt more "safe and secure from all alarms" than I had since my life fell apart when I got pregnant in 1943.

When I returned to our room after the service, Jarvis was still there. He had pulled his chair close to Wilma's armchair so he could hear her faint voice. I offered to try to find a wheelchair again, so we could take her outside on this beautiful sunny day. Soon we were strolling along the paved pathway, Jarvis pushing the chair and Wilma, head down, eyes darting from side to side trying to take it all in as she rolled along. We passed the stone chapel then, and Wilma moved her hand, signaling us to stop. We three admired the handiwork of the talented craftsman, the perfect archways, and the fine detail. He had since moved on to building low stone walls and additional creations, but the chapel remained his masterpiece. It was a favorite spot, and was used for prayers, funerals, and weddings.

After Jarvis went home, Wilma asked me to tell her all about the church service. I described it in detail, and she even sang the hymns with me. She said she used to play a red and white accordion, too, and it was still at the farm. She remembered the words of the songs better than I. She had gone to church weekly as a kid, until rheumatoid arthritis relegated her to the status of what they called a "shut-in".

I told Wilma about Ronnie Galley, and she laughed at my straightening him out.

"I wonder where he is now."

I wondered, too. The last time I saw him, we were saying goodbye to several of the boys from town who had joined up and were leaving on the train. We stood on the station platform as the train came in. Ronnie's mother was crying as he first hugged her, and then his dad. As he stepped up into the train car, he turned and waved to us all.

OUR DEFENDER

Wilma was kind enough to share her dresser. I didn't require much space, as most of my belongings were stored at Marj's house. Wilma's dresses from home were neatly folded and unused, in the bottom drawer. When I saw them, I got a bright idea and I went ahead with it without permission, which may have been a mistake.

The staff had altered Wilma's standard grey canvas dresses worn by all female patients, by splitting the garment from top to bottom down the back. It was then more or less draped over the front of her body and tucked in on the sides, resembling a stiff blanket thrown over her. From the moment I saw her, the seamstress in me wanted to improve that situation for her comfort and appearance.

Dr. Sanders told me that a growing number of patients were stepping out on day passes as part of the outpatient program. Patients continued to successfully integrate back into the community, and the day passes were small steps toward this goal.

It was arranged that Marj would take me to her home for a short afternoon visit. My plan, which I didn't explain to anyone except Wilma, was that I would alter her dresses on my sewing machine. I took them with me that day, and I did it my way, opening the dresses at the back, neatly hemming the edges, and adding string ties to close the back of the neck and at the waist. When Marj saw what I was up to, she said she didn't think it would be too far in the future until the patients would own their clothing, shoes, and private effects.

Wilma was eager to see what I had done and when we tried on one of her dresses, she looked pretty and comfortable, and was delighted to wear her clothing after all these years. I had no idea I had transgressed.

The following Sunday, we were waiting for Jarvis to come, when we heard his voice down the hall in the direction of the nurses' desk. Wilma was eager to surprise him by wearing a dress he would recognize from when she lived at home. Mrs. Davis usually worked on Sundays, but we realized this was her weekend off, and in her place was our least favorite nurse, Mrs. Ross. It was her voice we could hear arguing with Jarvis. The altercation was heated, and loud enough that we could hear word for word what was being said.

"Your sister is no better than the other patients in this hospital. She is required to wear the institutional clothing issued to her, and I personally will enforce that rule!"

Wilma and I were shocked to hear Jarvis reply in no uncertain terms. "There's where you're wrong, dead wrong!"

Mrs. Ross was just getting started. "Special privileges are not allowed, Mr. Sim. I've been waiting for you to walk in here, so I can set you straight once and for all. You need to know it's that roommate of hers who is responsible for this dress business. She'll be sent to the Women's Ward, where she belongs this afternoon and there'll be no further favors for favorite people! I'm putting a stop to it."

"You're out of line, Mrs. Ross. I am my sister's guardian and you will not dictate what clothing she wears. Dr. Sanders is in charge of these two patients. You need to pull in your horns!"

I had no idea that Jarvis could yell like that. He was the meekest, mildest man I had ever met. This was a new Jarvis Sim, and Wilma and I were snickering, probably because of the tension and for the sheer joy of being defended.

Mrs. Ross sounded composed when she added, "There are rules in this hospital, Mr. Sim."

"And you can just take your rules and stick them where the sun won't shine on them!"

At that, Wilma and I burst out laughing. We couldn't help it and we couldn't quit. No doubt we could be heard down the hallway, especially me, with my extra loud cackle, but we could not stop. We were like a pair of school girls. Every time we tried to get sober, we thought of Jarvis' last comment and we were gone again. Poor

Wilma was gasping for air. It gave new meaning to the phrase "to die laughing".

In a couple of minutes, Jarvis tapped on the door frame, as the door was already open. He smiled as if nothing had happened, as if he hadn't just had a rip-roaring fight with the supervisor of the ward! Seeing Wilma dressed in a light green dress with a lace collar, he shook his head, and pulled a chair close to her armchair. Still smiling, he touched her twisted hand, "You're pretty as a picture, Wilma."

We expected trouble later on, but as long as Jarvis was there, we were convinced he would keep a lid on things. As he left, I thought about the long walk and locked doors to the Women's Ward. I really would have no choice if they came for me. They didn't.

That night before bed, Wilma asked in her quiet voice, "Liz, where do you think Mrs. Ross put her rules?" I had to cover my head with my pillow to keep from waking the whole ward.

A SONG IN MY HEART

The hospital was different now. So many changes since those grim days in the '40s, when I spent my days feeling more like a prisoner than a patient. Activities were organized and scheduled on different days, suited for different skill levels. The handicraft sale was held twice a year, with quality items that were popular in the community. The sale brought in a large sum of money for the general coffers, and some of it was used to replenish the craft supplies.

I put my handwork skills to use so that I was personally contributing and paying for my keep. I mostly did embroidery and knitting, and as I stitched, I was thankful for Aunt Flo's painstaking lessons. She insisted I learn correctly, and made me practice until I was an expert. As she often said, "You don't want to make a balls of it."

I embroidered pillowcases, tablecloths, and hankies. I enjoyed knitting most of all: slippers, socks, mittens, and gloves. I designed my patterns, and somehow that satisfied my creativity. Every item I produced had my personal stamp on it, because there were no others like it.

I continued to marvel at the progressive changes in the hospital. I was asked to teach knitting, and the ones in my group were especially enthusiastic, as I kept the conversation going, and the radio on. I had my Knitting Club on Wednesdays, and Wilma came with me in a wheelchair. Although she was unable to knit, she enjoyed the company. Marj brought my radio from her place, which livened up our session, and kept us in the know as to the weather and local happenings in the community. No one objected when I cranked up the volume for the *Let's Go West* show in the afternoons. So, we had some toe-tapping knitters in my group. They were patients who didn't care a fig about knitting, but asked to join us because as they said, "Your group has the most fun!"

We all enjoyed the camaraderie, and Wilma made friends, the same as the rest of us. As the sale date approached, we began regular sewing days. A couple of sewing machines were installed in the activity room. It was a cooperative group effort, drawing participants out of their shells. Potholder pieces were cut out, pinned, and then sewn together at the treadle machines. Dishtowels were embroidered, some hemmed by machine and some by hand. Each of us began to feel a sense of belonging.

I remembered making necklaces from the berries on the wolf willow bushes that grew at the back of Aunt Flo's yard. They were also plentiful in all the pastures and ditches in the area. The Rogers girls and I picked buckets of them, and soaked them in water. Inside each berry was a hard oval-shaped brown seed with lengthwise yellow strips. They were very pretty once we cleaned them off, and we strung them on strong thread with colored glass beads between each seed. Wilma remembered doing the same when she was at home, and several other patients recalled making them in years gone by.

We asked Linda to bring berries from the farm, so we could provide novel merchandise for the craft sale. Even after being soaked in water, the seeds were tough, and we used a thimble to force the needle through. The result was some unique and very pretty jewelry that enhanced our display of items at the sale.

On a Saturday afternoon in mid-July, I was waiting for tea time to be announced. I had been asked to meet with some volunteers who were interested in learning how to make wolf willow necklaces to use as a craft with some patients. I was enjoying a moment of quiet before they arrived, and suddenly I had the shock of a lifetime.

It happened to be Mrs. Ross on duty who came up behind me, drummed me on the shoulder, and said, "Your nieces are here, Liz." She had not spoken to me since her argument with Jarvis, and she disappeared as quickly as she came.

I could hardly believe my eyes when Dot Cleaver stood in front of me saying ever so quietly, "Liz, it's me, Dot." Tears were streaming down her face. Oh, it was a comfort to wrap that little girl in my arms! Her stepmother was with her, pretty much a girl herself, and noticeably bent on soaking up every word of our conversation.

My visitors admitted they had lied at the nurses' desk, saying they were my nieces so they could readily get in to see me. That wouldn't have worked years ago, but the rules were slack now on 3C. All they had to do was sign the visitors' book, and record the time in and time out. We had a giggle over the girls fooling Mrs. Ross, and I told them she was the perfect one to play a prank on.

It was a relief to explain about my Graves' disease and that it had sneaked up on me. It was no one's fault, not theirs, and not mine. I could tell Dot already had forgiven me for leaving them, as she poured out her heart in the short time we had together. I was reminded of the Rogers kids when we played in the yard after school. A couple of them would have a fight. Inevitably, one kid would get hurt and the other would march off to the house, crying a warning, "I'm telling!" Dot needed to tell someone, and I was eager to listen.

She told about her dad getting married and not letting them know beforehand, and she was still boiling angry with him for being secretive about her mother's death. She said she hated him. If she remembers anything from our little talk, I hope she takes my advice to let it go. I told her I hated my dad, too, but I was careful not to burden her with the details. I told her there were lots of reasons to hate my dad but it was only hurting me. I could tell that struck a chord with her, because the tears spilled down her face again. I reached for her hand, and I said, "Let it go, Dot. Loving is easier than hating."

Our visit wasn't all sadness. She asked if I will get well again, and I told her I am fine if I take my medication. She chattered about school and told me that the salt and flour map of Canada we worked on scored 100% in the Saskatchewan Golden Jubilee school competition. When I asked about the boys, she said little Mac still sings the song, "Jambalaya" and Nicky continues to be obsessed with nature science. Will sewed the pajamas we had cut out and started when I was there, and Roy still has a crush on Louise Bell. I asked her to give them my love.

Our time together was short because their ride was expected one hour after they arrived. What a brave and endearing little girl! As I told her when she left me, the visit put a song in my heart. By this time, I had missed my meeting with the volunteers, so I hurried back to our room to see if Wilma had awakened from her afternoon nap. She would be excited to hear all about my special visitor.

SON OF A MOOSE

We were happy to see an increasing number of local volunteers join us for evening activities. I went to the gathering room, as a sing-a-long was planned, and they especially welcomed anyone who could hold a tune. I noticed an unfamiliar volunteer there, a fairly young woman, who attempted to conceal her nervousness with a wide smile.

Suddenly one of the patients, Allan Pickering, stood abruptly to his feet. He looked around as if he had forgotten something important, and yelled, "Son of a moose!" He headed for the door with a nurse close behind him. As for the rest of us, we were used to that sort of thing. There were a few snickers here and there as Allan had caught us off guard, but it was the most recent recruit who lost it. I know she wasn't laughing *at* Allan but she laughed so uncontrollably, I thought we might have to carry her out. At the end of the sing-a-long, I took some shortbread cookies off the lunch table for Wilma.

When we told Jarvis about it on Sunday, he smiled and said, "I know him. His farm was close to ours. I think I'll go have a little chat." When Jarvis returned, he said he and Allan had a good old-fashioned visit.

I had to explain. "When anything in here makes us laugh, it seems to be the right thing. Laughter is healing. I hope you don't think we were laughing *at* him, Jarvis."

"You don't ever have to worry about that, Liz. You, of all people, know and understand that we are equal human beings, living under the same sun and breathing the same air."

I thought about his words after he went home. I said to Wilma, "That brother of yours is a smart man."

"I know," she answered in her muffled voice. "He gets it from me!"

How Wilma managed to be cheerful, despite her physical state, I couldn't fathom. We were always getting a chuckle out of something. I remembered the times in my life when there was no humor whatsoever. I do not remember hearing one person laugh at the Home for Unwed Mothers, but I often heard the sound of girls crying in their beds at night.

One day, I was wheeling Wilma outside, when a grey-haired woman sitting on a bench held up her hand, motioning us to stop.

I greeted her with, "Hello, young lady."

She had a frown on her face. "I know how you can fix her," she said, staring at Wilma's twisted limbs.

"And how's that?" I asked.

"You can rub butter all over her."

I saw Wilma's shoulders shake a little, but I kept a straight face. "Butter! How will that help?"

"I don't know, but my doctor says that's what you should do."

Wilma was visibly shaking by this time.

"Well," I sighed, "it will take a lot of butter, as she's a tall girl."

"It will work, I guarantee it. The doctor said."

As the wheelchair rounded the next corner, I stopped, knelt beside Wilma, and we laughed our heads off.

FEAR NOT

K en, the round-faced preacher, was speaking in the gathering room on a Sunday afternoon. "The winds of adversity blow on every one of us at one time or another, and most of you have had more than your share."

I wondered just how much adversity this sheltered young man had experienced in his twenty-five or so years. Twyla was on the front row listening intently, although I suspect she had to sit through the same sermon in their church that morning.

I set out several chairs before they arrived, but less than a dozen patients straggled in during the singing. The hymn books were ignored by all except the three of us, Ken, Twyla, and I, and we worked our way through the old hymns, which they had chosen to fit the theme.

Ken lifted the accordion and set it on Twyla's knee, and she put her arms through the straps. For such a slight gal, she could play with gusto, and I enjoyed the music as I always did.

Allan Pickering had nodded off to sleep, slumped in his chair in front of me. Perhaps Jarvis could be persuaded to come next time and help keep Allan awake. Even though some of the folks slept through the whole thing, I acknowledged their good intention to come. By attending this little church service, we were reaching out for help.

I had already bought into Ken's analogy on the storms of life, and was making a personal comparison. The wind had blown me to "heck and gone" - to the Home for Unwed Mothers and to the Provincial hospital twice. I felt like a corked bottle, bouncing on the ocean waves, thither and yon.

Just before the sermon, Ken picked up his guitar and said, "Turn to page 120, "A Shelter in the Time of Storm."

The Lord's our Rock in Him we hide,
A shelter in the time of storm
Secure whatever ill betide,
A shelter in the time of storm

We listened to the Bible story of a vicious storm on the Sea of Galilee. It took only three magic words, "Peace be still", and the wind was instantly calm. Ken said, "Wouldn't we all love to have our storms miraculously disappear, just like that? Miracles do happen sometimes, but more often something else happens, a different kind of miracle. The storm doesn't disappear, but we are given enough strength to bear it."

"You've experienced that strength," Ken continued. "I have, too."

After the service, Allan woke up, as did the other sleepers, and Ken shook hands with each one as they left the room. I remained seated on my chair. Ken waited awhile, and then sat down beside me.

"A lot of storms, Liz." It was a statement, not a question.

I nodded. Twyla gathered the hymnbooks and stacked them in the box. Then she sat quietly nearby, probably praying for my soul. Ken was not pushy. I thought of Wilma's frequent comment, "Talk it out." I had nothing to hide.

I asked, "How much time do you have?"

He grinned. "All afternoon, and longer if need be." He motioned to his wife to come and join us. "Sit here, Twyla."

For better or for worse, I shared my story with this young couple, who seemed to be so much younger than I, but were willing to listen with compassion.

"Okay, I'll give you the short version. My mother died when I was a little child. That's when the adversarial winds began to blow. I had an abusive father, and that wind blew me into the arms of a loving guardian who sheltered me. The next storm was terrifying. I got pregnant when I was twenty, and I had no support. Like one hurricane quickly following another, I was immediately blown down by a condition known as Graves' disease. I lost my baby, and for awhile, I lost my sanity as well. I came to the hospital, and after years of living here, I worked my way out, only to be blown back in with a flare-up of the Graves' disease. So that's about it, up until now. I've talked through the issues with supportive friends, and I've come to terms with the past."

"Well done, Liz. You're moving forward."

"I stayed to talk to you because I'm afraid. I don't know when the next storm clouds will rumble, or where they will take me. I know change is coming. If I do get out of here, I may get smacked with Graves' again. I have a dream of helping unmarried mothers, but I'm stuck with an uncertain future of my own. Usually, I don't think about it. But sometimes, like today, it really gets me."

I liked Ken. He didn't pretend to be a fancy minister. He was like a neighbor boy next door, willing to be a friend.

"I missed something today, Liz. Something really important. Two words often come up in the Bible, 'Fear not.' Way more important than anything else I said today. When the storms come, we naturally are afraid, but the real message is 'fear not' because a loving God is with us, no matter what's ahead."

Ken said a prayer for me. I felt the love. Somewhere in the depths of my being, I let the fear go. Twyla, who had said nothing throughout the whole event, held my hand for a moment, and said in her quiet little voice, tears in her eyes, "God knows your dreams."

It was a perfect way to end. We said goodbye at the door and I hurried back to Wilma, eager to tell her about the service and my experience. I met Jarvis just outside our room.

He showed his surprise. "Liz! What the heck happened to you? Your face is positively shining."

"I've got peace in my soul, Brother Sim!" Poor Jarvis never could tell if I was serious or not. This time I was.

FOR THE LOVE OF
A STRANGER

For four days, Wilma and I were glued to the radio in our room. The Springhill Mine disaster in Nova Scotia occurred on Thursday evening, Nov. 1. From that moment on, Wilma and I were part of the throng of friends and families waiting at the mine entrance for news. We grieved the death of the ones who were already gone, and we anxiously listened hour by hour for news of the men trapped below. By Saturday afternoon, the announcement came down from top officials. There was no hope for survivors. The debris and toxic gases made rescue impossible, and a decision was imminent to seal the mine. We were heartsick when we heard it.

But the rescuers weren't willing to stop. They risked their lives as they pressed down deeper and deeper with ventilation equipment and expertise, determined not to give up.

On Sunday afternoon, I skipped the church service I usually attended, so we could continue our vigil by the radio. Jarvis arrived as usual at two o'clock and joined Wilma and me in our concern and conversation regarding the Springhill miners.

As we later learned, two groups of men were trapped with limited air supply. Seven brave miners in the deepest area crawled through to the first group, stopping at every air valve, gasping for a breath of oxygen as they continued on. They worked their way upward, knowing it was life or death for them all. Those heroes proved to be tougher than the coal they had been mining all their lives. At 3500 feet, they met the rescuers and the rest is history!

Jarvis, who usually went home in the later afternoon, stayed with us until well after dark, when word came through that the deepest cluster of men had been reached. Wilma cried as emotional news reporters thousands of miles to the east assured us that every miner would be out by Monday morning.

When it was all over, and the death toll tallied, 39 had died in the disaster; 88 survived. I wondered why we cared so much about those strangers we would never meet. Perhaps crisis in our own lives sharpened our sensitivity for the plight of others. Maybe it was simply a clearer understanding of those memorable words Jarvis said about Allan Pickering, "We are all equal human beings, living under the same sun, and breathing the same air."

PLEASE DON'T SAY IT

During one of my weekly visits to Dr. Sander's office towards the end of March, he opened a topic I didn't want to hear.

"I've spoken with Wilma and with her brother and they've given me permission to speak to you." I wondered what this was all about. My heart sank. Surely, he wasn't going to move me to another room!

"You need to know that Wilma's health is declining, and there is not a lot we can do for her."

Before he said another word, I protested, "But she's only 44 years old! That's too young."

I thought quickly of Aunt Flo and her congestive heart failure. She wasn't really old, but not young like this.

Dr. Sanders continued. "Only the Man Upstairs knows the future, Liz. I hope to be wrong, but I feel I should prepare you. She may leave us sooner than we think."

"But have you tried everything? There must be..."

Dr. Sanders interrupted me. "You should see her thick file, Liz. She's endured every imaginable treatment. Bed rest was the initial prescribed remedy, then iron via IV, and the gold treatments with very harsh side effects. She's even had casts on her joints. In 1953, there was a buzz in the medical world touting cortisone as a cure, but there's no cure for RA. The best treatment of all is the love and care she received from her family, and now from you."

The tears welled up. It was Dr. Sanders who had explained to me long ago, after my surgery, that it was expected I would be calmer, and less emotional than normal. I found that to be true and I referred to myself, proudly as, "Liz, the woman who never cries." It was less embarrassing to be in control of my tears. At Dr. Sander's suggestion that Wilma would leave us, I felt an instant lump in my throat. She was like a sister to me, a friend who had seen me through healing from my past, a listener like no other.

The doctor reminded me, "One way to look at it is from Wilma's view. Those swollen, inflamed joints cause her pain every waking moment. She has extreme fatigue. She has a wonderful attitude and outlook, but she's tired. The pain exhausts her."

I knew that. I had been thinking just now of all she was to me, and how I couldn't do without her. He turned my attention now to Wilma's pain and endurance.

"But she's not depressed," I countered.

"I don't believe she is either. I'm just giving you a heads up, Liz. Her heart is very weak. It has been a joy and an inspiration to see the mutual friendship forged between the two of you. I'm hoping, too, that it lasts for a long while yet."

I left his office sad and somber. Nothing lasts forever. Not the good, and not the bad. Dr. Sanders was right. How could I have been so blind? It had been a long while since Wilma had asked for my help so she could stand and look out the window. Her meals took way longer now, and she went to sleep earlier at night. She slept longer in the afternoon, except on Sundays when Jarvis came.

I determined to make every day count. We talked a lot when she was able. We invited Linda and her mom in for afternoon tea. Jarvis now came twice a week. Even on a stormy day, we would suddenly hear a tap on the door and see him there, with a smile for his sister. When Linda came, she talked non-stop about Bob, her "steady Freddy" and how funny he was. She said he just made her laugh all the time. I noticed her mother did not comment on the boyfriend.

NO PLACE TO GO

Wilma and many others at the hospital were not there for mental illness issues. It was a catch-all center for those who had no place to go for care that was beyond family help at home.

Early on a Sunday afternoon, I pushed Wilma's wheelchair outside for a pleasant walk around the grounds. We preferred the smooth paved path towards the parking lot, and it was there we encountered a middle-aged lady, weeping, with a white handkerchief covering most of her face.

When we met her on the walkway. I stopped, and for lack of a better choice of words, I simply said, "I'm sorry."

She cried even more as I waited, and then she asked, "Can't you do something?"

I immediately realized she mistook me for staff as I probably appeared to be Wilma's attendant. Since the hospital had finally discarded those awful grey dresses, we had worn all those years, our status as a patient was probably not now as recognizable to a stranger.

The woman poured out her story. Her father was 77 years old and in fine health, until a sudden stroke in the past week took him to the hospital. Since the stroke, his speech was slurred, and his right side partially paralyzed.

"They say this is the only place for him now. But he's begging me to take him home. I can't take it."

"You can't manage his care, can you?"

"No, that's just the thing. I couldn't possibly lift him, and we don't have a bathroom in our house on the farm."

I looked closely at her face, a much older woman now, but I recognized her from my childhood in Cala.

"Are you Rita Coleman?"

133

She raised her head sharply to look me in the eye, "Liz. It's you, Liz Parker. Of course, I remember you. Are you working here now?"

"No Rita, I'm a patient."

"Really? Not you, Liz. I didn't know."

"I remember your dad, too."

"They say he's *violent*! My dad has never been violent in his life. He's just confused and wants to get out."

"I know that feeling. I know it well."

I understood my place as a patient at the hospital. I was well aware that I may be overstepping my boundaries, but people are people. I put my arms around Rita and she sobbed on my shoulder.

"Some of the nurses are kind and caring," I said, hoping to be of comfort. I was in particular thinking of Mrs. Davis, who meant so much to Wilma and me.

"Well, I sure haven't met them yet," Rita said. She glanced at her truck parked nearby.

"Come often, Rita. Even though it's hard for you, it will mean everything to him."

Rita appeared to be overwhelmed that she had met someone she knew. Perhaps it helped her perspective to see that I was now a patient, and that Wilma was transported in a wheelchair, unable to raise her head. Rita's crisis was hard to bear, but she was not alone. There is a lot of suffering.

"Thank you, Liz, thanks so much."

We watched her go. Somewhere across town, a Sunday afternoon ballgame would be in full swing, with a crowd cheering and laughing. Customers would stop at the Tastee Freeze window to order fish and chips or soft ice cream, or maybe a float for fifteen cents. When your heart is filled with pain, it's unthinkable that others are glibly passing the day with trivialities. During some of my deepest, loneliest, and most depressing moments, I was aware of a hearty laugh, perhaps a couple of nurses sharing a joke, and I would think, "How can you laugh? I'm dying, and you are laughing."

I pushed the wheelchair towards the chapel where the flowerbeds were bursting with a riot of color. I bent down close to Wilma so she could hear me from her folded position.

"What are your thoughts, my friend?" I asked.

Believing her brother could walk on water, her reply was barely audible. "Let's see if Jarvis can go visit Rita's father."

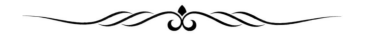

LEAVING THE
PAST BEHIND

After seeing Rita Coleman from the town where I was raised, my mind kept wandering back to that community, and to the folks I had known there. The Rogers family had made an indelible print on me, as they were my siblings after a fashion. We played games till late at night in the summer. Hide and Seek in the dark was a favorite. We lit bonfires and we explored the outskirts of town, making memories that didn't matter, but they made up our childhood. Mrs. Rogers was always kind and welcoming to me, I think mostly because I didn't mind looking after the little kids. I told them stories when she was too busy to keep track of them. Mulling over the past was making me unusually quiet, and Wilma questioned me.

"What's buzzing in that billion-dollar brain of yours?"

"Oh, I'm revisiting the past again. I think I do that too often lately."

Wilma said, "I wander down memory lane a lot myself, and I don't think it does me any harm."

Wilma was a listener like no other. "Talk it out," was her common suggestion to me. I told her there was something I was pondering, something I had never told another living soul. I could see her smiling down into the folds of her pretty purple dress. Then she said, "Talk it out, Liz. I'm here!"

And so, I shared with Wilma what happened the night before I got in my brother's car and sped away from my beloved home in Cala that chilly early morning in October of 1943.

Ralph had arrived late in the evening, and Aunt Flo told me to fix up a bed for him in the living room. The couch was still there, as the people hadn't come for it yet, but we no longer had extra sheets. I used two blankets, one for the top and one for the bottom, and gave him a pillow off my bed. We would be leaving early in the morning for the Home for Unwed Mothers, and so he had to spend the night.

It would be my last night in my room, my final goodbye to our house, and to our town, and to my childhood. I slipped out the door, and wandered to the shed at the back of our property. I remembered with thanks that the sale of old Bally's milk had helped us through the Dirty Thirties. Chickens were roosting on their poles inside the shed, and the younger Rogers kids were slated to collect them before Aunt Flo left the property on the weekend.

It was late, and there were no stars. The yard was familiar, so I easily found my way in the dark. I leaned on the rail fence between our yard and Rogers' property. That's when I heard a familiar voice. It was Carl.

"I was hoping you might be out here. I wanted to talk to you before you go."

When Carl found out a few weeks prior that I was pregnant, he told me what he would like to do to Ray Hutton, which included a beating and a surgical procedure with a rusty knife. I appreciated his loyalty, but couldn't help but think, "Men! Their first solution is always to settle a problem with their fists!"

"Liz, I have a proposition for you. I think we should get married."

I half-laughed, half-choked,

"Hear me out. I've got two options, and I need you to help me choose. Remember my Grandpa Rogers on the farm north of town?"

I nodded, wondering where this was going.

"He's really old and frail now. The drought nearly took him out. He's offered me the farm."

"Oh Carl, you lucky duck!"

Farming had long been a dream of mine. I loved the times I had stayed overnight on a farm with a friend from school. Even as a kid back then, I was sure the work would suit me. Everything about country living appealed to me: a huge garden, the animals, and the birds. The pastureland and the fields were so much bigger than our postage stamp sized lot in town.

I had respect and admiration for the Saskatchewan pioneers like Carl's grandfather, who had come forty years before, and carved out a new life on the prairie. I loved their spirit and their determination to make it, side by side, with fellow settlers in the area.

Carl touched my arm. "Liz, marry me. We can take over his farm."

I stared at him in disbelief. He continued his campaign.

"I missed out on the war, but when the boys come home with nothing but stories of guns and the Eiffel Tower, I'll be sitting pretty on my own farm! But that's only if we do it together. If I settle out there now, I'll be the one-eyed bachelor farmer for the rest of my life."

I felt detached from what Carl was proposing. "What's your other choice, Carl?"

"I can head down east. The army will take me, along with the guys they turned down. A lot of women work there, too, in Ontario, at the munitions factory. It's a job, and a way of contributing to the war effort. So, I have two choices Liz, but my preference is to take over the farm with you."

I saw Carl's offer for what it was. It was a one-minute-to-midnight offer. There was no time for logical consideration, or to talk it over with my aunt. This was a chicken way out, a cobbled-together plan, based on convenience and need, some of each for both of us.

"I'm thinking of you, too, Liz. It's not going to be easy with a baby on your own."

"I know that Carl, but it's not your baby."

I saw a flash of hurt cross his face. "You think that matters? You know our family better than that by now, Liz. At our house, a baby is a baby. I would never play favorites."

I had never once thought of loving Carl as a boyfriend, let alone a husband. Ruth and I called each other sisters, just for fun. She would be elated if such a thing came true. My mind was racing, Carl was serious.

"Carl, I've always loved you and Ruth, and the rest of your family. I'm like a sister to you. You couldn't love me as a wife."

Even in the dark, I could tell he was smiling. "Yes, I could, in the blink of an eye!" Carl was known for joking about his loss of vision. He had just said "in the blink of an eye", but neither of us laughed.

"It just doesn't feel right."

"I won't beg you, Liz."

He put his arms around me. Carl Rogers, my friend, and my brother since we were eight years old.

"It wouldn't be fair, Carl, not to any one of the three of us." When he hugged me, I felt the baby between us.

"Good luck, Liz. If you need me..."

I crept into the house, and to my room for the last sleep in the tall bed that wasn't so tall anymore. I stared at the ceiling most of the night. By morning, I still didn't know if I should get in Ralph's car, or if I should run as fast as I could across the yard to the Rogers' house. Right or wrong, I had to go with my good sense.

Wilma heard my story. After a long pause, she said almost inaudibly. "I don't think there really is a right or wrong, Liz. We need to make the best choice we can at the time, and then live with the results."

We both loved the 1956 Doris Day release, "Que Sera, Sera". Every time the song came on the radio, and that was often, I sang along, thinking of my roller coaster life events. What if I could have been a farmer's wife? What if Wilma had not been derailed by rheumatoid arthritis? So many "what ifs". After telling Wilma about Carl's proposal, I was finally able to put those thoughts to rest, and leave them in the past where they belonged.

WILMA'S STORY

Wilma described her unbearable early days at the hospital. She was admitted in 1950, the same year I became an outpatient. We were like ships passing in the dark.

Her mother had lovingly cared for her throughout the years, as rheumatoid arthritis steadily robbed her daughter of the ability to care for herself. Wilma had never lived away from home, nor had she ever been separated from her family. When her mother died suddenly, there was no time to prepare or plan for the future. The only option for Wilma was the Saskatchewan Hospital.

"Jarvis would have moved heaven and earth for me but the one thing he couldn't do was be my nursemaid. When he brought me to the hospital, we cried all the way to the city. As he drove on to the bridge, I told him it was time to buck up and make our mother proud of us."

The first weeks were the worst, even though at the beginning Jarvis made the 29-mile trip each and every day. Wilma longed for her home. She missed the home cooking, the quiet peaceful farm sounds, birds in the morning, chatting with her brother, and most of all, she missed her mother. At home, Jarvis had carried her from room to room, to a bed they had set up outside, and to the car for a ride to town when she felt up for it. In the hospital, she was stuck in one place and was controlled by the inflexible schedule. I realized Wilma's sudden admittance to the hospital was similar to mine, with near-impossible adjustments to make.

"Tell me about your mom."

"Oh Mom? She was a great woman! She had a Scottish accent, and she did a lot of singing around the house. That's why I love to hear you singing as you do, with the radio, or on your own. It reminds me of her."

"What songs were her favorites?"

"She sang the old songs, like "Bicycle Built for Two", "Put on Your Old Gray Bonnet", those ones."

I remembered them from the yellow song sheet in Mr. Peter's class. Just for fun, I started to clap and sing.

> *Put on your old grey bonnet with the blue ribbon on it,*
> *While I hitch old Dobbin to the shay.*
> *And through the fields of clover, we'll drive up to Dover*
> *On our golden wedding day.*

Wilma burst out laughing.

"What's so funny?"

"I just remembered one time when Mom nearly shocked Jarvis out of his skin. She was very much a serious-minded lady, but one morning I woke up with my joints acting up. Because I was having a hard time, she must have been trying to cheer me up. She was cooking breakfast, but she grabbed Jarvis' felt hat from the coat hook by the door and pulled it down nearly over her eyes. She pranced around the stove like a horse, and lit into singing, *"Put on your old grey bonnet with the blue ribbon on it, while I hitch old Dobbin to the shay"*.

Just then Jarvis came in from doing chores. He stood there, with his hand on the doorknob and his mouth hanging wide open. As if Mom weren't wearing his hat and pretending to be old Dobbin in the song, she said as normal as could be, "Say, Lad, will you fetch me some wood? I'm making panny-cakes for breakfast."

It still makes me laugh. He was so surprised, and so was she."

We loved the story. I could pretty well imagine it.

"There's another song Mom liked to sing. It was called "Twilight Is Falling". Do you know that one, too?"

I nodded. "I do." I sang the first line, *"Twilight is falling over the sea."*

The next time Jarvis came, Wilma asked if we could sing it. She was sure Jarvis would remember the words. He did, and so the three of us sang the chorus together.

Far away beyond the starlit skies,
Where the love light never, never dies,
Gleameth a mansion filled with delight,
Sweet happy home so bright.

At the end of the song, we were quiet. Then Wilma said, "See Jarvis, I told you Liz sings just like Mom."

It had become a struggle to help Wilma get into bed. She and I had a system, but it took some time to do it safely, especially as she required more support than before.

Jarvis said, "I'll lift you into bed, Wilma, like I used to."

I quickly pulled back the covers, and he gently placed her in the middle of the bed. I could feel the love between them. I was happy they'd had such a dedicated mother, who would be proud of them, as Wilma had hoped.

WE'LL SAY GOODNIGHT
HERE BUT GOOD
MORNING UP THERE

On June 28th, I woke up as usual at 6:30 in the morning. I called "Good morning" across the room, as Wilma was always awake before I was. Usually, she moved her hand in a sort of way to reply, as her voice was not strong, especially when she was lying down. Her hands were still. I knew instinctively that Wilma *was* having a good morning, but she was not here.

I dressed quickly and was relieved to see it was Mrs. Davis on shift at the nurses' desk.

I said, "She's gone."

Mrs. Davis quickly came around to the front of the desk and squeezed my hand.

"Are you okay, Liz?"

My heart felt so heavy in my chest, I thought I couldn't bear it. "Can I tell Jarvis?"

"Yes, of course. That's best. I'll put a long-distance call through."

In a minute or two, I heard him say hello. I hadn't planned what I would say. So it just came out, "Jarvis, our girl is gone."

The hospital had a morgue, and the funeral was held two days later. Friends and neighbors living near their farm home attended, as well as some of the staff. We barely fit into the little stone chapel.

I had asked Jarvis if Ken and Twyla could come and do the music. He said he would arrange whatever I wanted. There was a prayer to begin, and I had chosen three hymns, accompanied by the preacher's guitar. The old songs gave me comfort. "What a Friend We Have in Jesus", and "Leaning on the Everlasting Arms".

I decided to tackle the third song as a solo. I don't know where the courage came from, but I needed to sing the song Wilma and Jarvis remembered their mother singing, the same one we sang together only a couple of Sunday nights before.

Twilight is falling over the sea,
Shadows are falling dark on the lee.
Born on the night winds voices of yore,
Come from that far off shore.

I had no idea if I would fall flat on my face and ruin the service, or if I would take it over the top. With that uncertainty, I joined Ken at the front of the chapel. He didn't know the song, but it helped that he was chording along on his guitar. From the opening note, I knew it was going to be okay. Never had I been happier that my singing voice returned after my thyroid surgery.

Far away beyond the starlit skies,
Where the love light never, never dies.
Gleameth a mansion filled with delight,
Sweet happy home so bright.

Jarvis sat with his head bent, looking down at his feet during most of the service, but he looked up during those words. I hoped it meant something special to him. It was a tough day for a devoted brother.

The elderly minister, Rev. Bergen, took over the rest of the service. He had been acquainted with the family for years. He had conducted funeral services for both their parents, and had known Wilma since she was a child. Linda's mom helped Jarvis write a tribute, and Rev. Bergen read it after the hymns.

"Wilma Eleanor Sim was born April 10, 1913, and was raised on the family farm five miles east of Tansy. Wilma was a quiet, gentle girl who loved children, animals, and music. She attended the Tansy

Hills School until she was diagnosed with rheumatoid arthritis at age 13, when she was forced to bed rest at home, and to give up her pursuit of playing the accordion and painting.

She was a brave and kind woman who did not complain about her relentless pain or her limitations. She made this world a brighter place. She is deeply missed by her best friend and roommate, Liz Parker, and by her loving brother, Jarvis Sim."

At the end of the service, the group walked to the cemetery on the grounds. Ken and Twyla were beside me.

Twyla said, "Your song was beautiful, Liz. Perfect for Wilma." The sky was overcast. The world was a poorer, darker place without the warmth and courage of Wilma Sim.

I saw the neighbors shaking hands with Jarvis in the parking lot before they drove away. Mrs. Davis and I returned to the ward. My room was so empty. Wilma's bed had been removed, and only her armchair remained by the window.

Mrs. Davis brought a tray with a cup of tea and cookies, and then sat in the armchair for a few minutes. What I liked most about her was that she didn't force conversation. We sat there peaceful and thoughtful, taking a moment to let the loneliness fill the empty spaces in the room. There was a familiar tap on the door frame, and to my surprise, there was Jarvis. He hadn't gone home after all. Mrs. Davis stood to her feet.

"Sit down Jarvis. I'll get you a cup of tea, or would you rather coffee?"

Jarvis didn't protest. "I think coffee, please."

As always, I was first to speak, blurting out. "I loved her."

Jarvis quoted the old saying, "Better to have loved and lost than never to have loved at all." It was so appropriate. I wouldn't have traded the past year sharing this room with Wilma for anything.

Mrs. Davis brought his coffee and left. He stirred in cream and sugar.

"So you came in to say goodbye." He had come to this hospital once a week since 1950. Seven years! Every Sunday without fail, and more often recently, since Dr. Sanders sounded the alarm.

"No, not goodbye, Liz. On the contrary."

What he said next hit me like a ton of bricks. I didn't see it coming, not in a million years.

"You shouldn't be here Liz. I'd like to take you home with me. I've talked to Dr. Sanders about it, and I can sign you out as my housekeeper."

"Oh Jarvis, please don't think you owe me for taking care of Wilma! Whatever I did for her, I did for love, and you owe me nothing!"

"It's not for Wilma, it's for me." I saw how sad he was. Having me around would maybe in a small way, make him feel like Wilma was still present.

"I'm in shock."

"I've had this in my mind for a long time. It's time you got out. I'm asking you to consider it."

This was a lot to ponder. Of course, I couldn't talk it over with Wilma, but my faithful friend, Marj, was never far away. I would ask her advice, and together we would make a sensible decision.

When Jarvis finished his coffee, he smiled with his eyes. I knew his heart was aching as he left Wilma's chair.

"I'll come again tomorrow. You can sleep on the idea and let me know."

I followed him to the door, and watched him go towards the parking lot. I asked Mrs. Davis if I could use the phone to call Marj.

AS SURE AS THE RIVER

We stood beside the truck on that momentous summer day in July, only one week after the funeral. Jarvis had spent the past hour in the Main office, and as we went out the door, he carried my discharge papers in one hand, and my little brown suitcase in the other. It was the same suitcase I took to the Home for Unwed Mothers 14 years before. Somehow it had followed me from there to the Saskatchewan Hospital and vanished in the depths of some deep storage room. I wondered why they didn't give it to me when I went to Marj's as an outpatient.

He put the suitcase in the truck box close to the cab, and opened the door for me. I wasn't in a hurry to get in. I looked back at the tree-lined road, the profusion of multi-colored flowers, and the vast complex of brick buildings. I had spent a large portion of my life within those walls. Jarvis was patient.

Without looking at him, I made my request. "Please, make me a promise, Jarvis. Promise you'll bring me back if this doesn't work out. Don't let me make a fool of myself if I go haywire like I did at Cleaver's last year. Just bring me back here."

We were leaning on the passenger side of the truck box, and the door was still open for me. His arms were crossed, and he was listening intently as he always did.

"I'm taking you away from here, Liz, and I don't plan to bring you back, except for check-ups with the doctor." We had talked it over already. As I was not a relative, he had signed me out as his housekeeper, and was taking responsibility for me.

Jarvis talked slowly, which calmed me down when I was anxious. "I saw Dr. Sanders again just now. We've set it up. Every month, I'll bring you in for your appointment. They'll do tests to make sure your thyroid medication is working, and figure out if any treatment is needed. Your health will be our number one concern."

I couldn't take my eyes off the river. That scene had become part of my life. Every morning when I started work, and at lunchtime, I took a moment to look out the west windows, and again in the evening as the sun set on the water. The river was high from the June rains in the mountains, and was flowing swiftly, totally covering the sandbar that was usually visible in summer.

Jarvis had more to say. "I told the doctor I'll be staying with you when you come to see him. There won't be any surprises, Liz, you're not their property."

"Nothing's for sure, Jarvis. Nothing ever stays the same."

Later, I thought a lot about what he said next, "The river does."

By now, I was wise enough not to count one hundred percent on anything. We would see if something unforeseen robbed me of the present dream I had been offered. For now, I could only trust in Jarvis and his pure intentions. He would do his best to make this work, and I would, too.

"Fear not." Two words came to mind, and gave me the courage to take the plunge. When I finally slid onto the leather seat, Jarvis closed the passenger door and I looked straight ahead. So this was it - leaving again, at long last! We took the road toward the bridge. The well-kept hospital grounds grew smaller and smaller in the side mirror. This was my first ride in his truck, and I asked him the make and year. He seemed pleased that I was interested.

"1956 Chev.

"I like it." It was a bright shade of yellow.

"Remember last year I asked what your favorite color was? You said yellow. Well, that's when I bought the truck."

"You're kidding. I remember now. You asked us both and Wilma said purple."

"I remember that, too. I couldn't stand the thought of a purple truck, even if they made such a thing!"

By this time, the hospital was far behind us, and there was a mix of emotions going on in my head. Talking was my way of letting off the pressure.

"You know, I always thought if I got out permanently, I'd find a way to be a volunteer like the ones who were so uplifting to Wilma and me. In the last while though, I've changed my mind on that."

Jarvis nodded. Oh, this man was easy to talk to.

"I don't want to come back. They've got enough volunteers. There's something else, something I can't get off my mind."

Jarvis kept his eyes on the road. "Well, let's hear it! I never know what you'll come up with."

"I'm thinking about unwed mothers. I'd like to help set them back on their feet. I think about them a lot, those single pregnant girls."

"Were you one, Liz?"

There were so many things he didn't know about me. For a few seconds, I heard again the director's voice belittling and bullying me and threatening to take my baby.

"I was - a long time ago - and there wasn't a soul on earth who stood up for me."

THE GUEST HOUSE

When I moved to the farm, I asked Jarvis if I could snoop out-side. He was amused and said, "Of course". I could check out anything I wanted to. He assured me there were no dangers such as an open well to watch out for.

I felt like a kid back in my home town. Back then, on a Saturday afternoon after our chores were done, the neighbor kids and I went exploring. We rummaged through abandoned houses and empty sheds in the area. Old junk piles yielded special treasures that no one wanted, except us. I found an old lantern, cleaned it up, and filled it with coal oil. I used it when I went out to check the cow and the chickens at night.

Linda came into the yard as I was reminiscing and wandering from one building to another near the barn. We were soon walking and chatting together. I was grateful to already have a friend in my new surroundings. She was a bubbly teenager with her life full of plans and promises. Always, there was talk of Bob, her steady boy-friend, and their drive-in movie dates. She said she wanted me to meet him, because she was certain we would like each other.

The most appealing building out there was different from the other sheds and outbuildings. It looked like a miniature house, with windows and a smaller sized door. Inside, there were two bunks and a wood-burning airtight heater, hooks on the wall, and a couple of wooden chairs.

Linda spoke up. "I think this was a bunkhouse for a hired man. I remember seeing him once years ago, when Mom and I came to visit Wilma." Then we got talking about Linda's mom being a nurse, and how she had helped out with Wilma's care when she first got sick.

"I was the tag-a-long and Wilma took a liking to me. I'm not sure why. I was an active kid, always bouncing around, but she didn't mind. I probably brought some life into her confined world. She showed me how to draw, and I used to sing while she played the accordion. That was, of course, when she still had use of her hands, and needed some diversions. Mom often sent me over to visit Wilma, and that's how we became friends."

The bunkhouse intrigued me. After Linda left, I got a broom, a mop, and hot soapy water. A plan was taking shape in my head, and it was so freeing to know I could do whatever I wanted out here. There were no rules on the farm, no schedule, no restrictions. Jarvis had been out by the gas barrels filling the tractor. Before he left the yard, he came over and asked if I had found anything that caught my fancy.

"I sure did! Can I have this little house?"

He was always amused by my enthusiasm for something he would see as nothing.

"It's all yours Liz, to have and to hold."

I transformed the old bunkhouse into a sweet little home. I cleaned out all the old junk, and bought some new furniture. It was a thrill to use my own money that Ralph returned to me, for those purchases. I can't explain what it felt like to go buy something, and to have a place to put it. The hospital life was so restrictive. It was like I never really belonged there. Jarvis said I didn't, and I now believed him. This was home, right here on the farm, home sweet home.

I sewed curtains and a matching tablecloth. I painted the walls, inside and out. We added a small cook stove, and I filled the window sills with blooming houseplants. It was a dollhouse, and I loved to go sit there in the afternoons and have a cup of tea. Jarvis helped cut the grass around the outside of it and made a boardwalk path to the door. Some cowboy had nailed spurs and horseshoes to the outside wall by the door. We took those down. They might have been okay for a bunkhouse, but not for this little home.

We called it the guest house. Though we were unsure as to who would be our guest, it would be ready when the time came. I often thought of Twyla's quiet promise back at the hospital, "God knows your dreams."

I liked to take afternoon coffee and a snack to Jarvis when he was working in the field. I made sure to ask where he would be working, so I could find him. One day, there was a red tail hawk perched on a tall fence post, not far from where we had our lunch. I had seen it a couple of times before, and was surprised it didn't fly away when I showed up.

"He minds his own business, and so do I," Jarvis said with a grin. "We get along fine."

"Okay, what's his business, and what's yours?"

"Well, he's watching for mice, and I'm watching for you coming across the field."

BLUE SKIRT WALTZ

Acouple of weeks after I moved to the farm, I was sitting in Wilma's chair on a Saturday afternoon, paging through the Eaton's summer catalogue. The book stayed open as I admired all six dresses featured on the same page. The one marked "J" caught my eye. $8.98. Jarvis insisted on paying housekeeper wages, and for a moment, I thought I just might haul off and order it. I usually sewed my clothes, and hadn't bought any for a long while. I came to my senses immediately, as I had no place to wear such a pretty dress, and I would likely feel foolish in it. Jarvis was looking over my shoulder.

"Which one do you like?"

I was kidding him when I asked, "Well, which one do *you* like?"

He said, "The blue with the flowers." That was "J". I thought no more about it. The next Saturday afternoon he came in from town and put the groceries on the table for me to put away, and then handed me a package with the Eaton's red and white return address on it. I tore open the parcel. I shook out the dress and it was even prettier than pictured in the catalogue.

"What's this all about?" I asked, purely puzzled.

"I think it will suit you - try it on."

After supper dishes were done, I tried on the dress, and it was a fit! I sat there feeling like a queen on my throne, not wanting to take it off just yet. I checked through the collection of LPs beside the portable record player in the living room. They included several artists I liked and had enjoyed throughout the years, wherever I had lived.

I selected one I hadn't heard for quite a while. It was Frankie Yankovic and the "Blue Skirt Waltz". I thought Jarvis was still outside, but he appeared from nowhere and took a mock bow. And then we were dancing in the kitchen. It felt like the most natural thing in the world. I liked the fit and the feel of the blue dress. I still couldn't believe Jarvis had bought it for me.

He asked something he had never mentioned before, "So you never married, Liz?"

"No, not even once," I said with a smile. It was true for both of us. Not even once. As we circled the small space, the "Blue Skirt Waltz" matched my dress and my mood. I remembered the night Jarvis came to the volunteers' dance when Wilma was still with us. He was a good dancer.

"Jarvis, tell me why you never married."

Without missing a dance step, he explained, "I was too shy, that's all there was to it. There was a girl I had known from school, Verna Sinclair. I knew she liked me. One Saturday night, I went to a dance held at a school not far from here. I usually took my fiddle because I got paid a few dollars to play, but that meant I didn't get to dance."

I commented, "So it was money or love, and you had a choice?"

"No, it wasn't that. Simply this - on that particular night, Verna suddenly showed up beside me. The moment I took a breath to ask her to dance, along came an acquaintance. I stood there like an awkward schoolboy as she waltzed away. She looked at me over his shoulder, and her eyes were begging me to 'cut in'."

"And you were too shy?" I continued humming along with Frankie Yankovic.

Jarvis nodded. "I shoulda cut in."

I have never been short of words. "But just think, instead of Verna Sinclair, here you are waltzing with me in your kitchen to the tune of the 'Blue Skirt Waltz'."

I was tall, but Jarvis was taller. He smiled down at me, his brown eyes crinkling up on the edges. "You're absolutely right! Verna Sinclair, be hanged!"

I leaned my head on his shoulder. The waltz was over, the music ended, one last twirl, and a swish of the blue skirt. We sat down on either side of the table.

Jarvis was smiling his quiet, shy smile. "Thank you for the dance."

"You are very welcome."

After a quick cup of tea, I headed to my bed in the housekeeper room. Before I fell asleep, I had to grin into the darkness, and I said out loud, "Verna Sinclair, be hanged!"

In the morning I was awake early, gathered the eggs, and had breakfast ready when Jarvis came to the kitchen. There was warmth in the air, as we relived the memory of last night. Jarvis sat down at the table.

Always the talker of the two of us, I spoke first, "If someone peeked in this window last night, what do you think they saw? I bet they would have laughed at this odd couple waltzing around like a pair of kids."

Jarvis smiled and I continued my musing. "They would have seen a tall, lanky cowboy with a knack for dancing, but they'd have no way of seeing that you are a gentleman with a heart of gold."

Jarvis nodded, accepting the compliment.

"And they would have seen a woman with bug eyes, wearing a beautiful blue dress." Here Jarvis interrupted me, and took up the rest of my story.

"They couldn't have known they were looking at the kindest woman in the world who asks nothing for herself."

I saw then that he loved me, as plain as day. I could see it in his eyes. What happened next caught me by surprise. I felt the tide welling up somewhere deep within me. I managed only the words, "And they wouldn't have known they were looking at Liz, the lady who never cries."

Jarvis saw it coming one moment before I did. He settled me on his knee and folded me in his arms. He pressed my cheek against his rough, plaid shirt collar just in time. The dam burst. I cried and I cried, till the coffee boiled over on the stove and minutes passed without a word between us. I cried for the little girl I once was with no mama, and a deranged father. And for the cruelty and disdain at the hand of the director at the Home for Unwed Mothers. I cried for the baby girl I loved and lost, for the pain and the surgery and the humiliation of Graves' and the years on Ward 3C. I cried for Wilma, my forever friend who gave me purpose and helped me heal. I cried for the Cleaver kids back on the farm in McKeen where I had given my best and ruined it all at the end. Most of all, I cried for this man, this angel of a man who was holding me, loving me for no reason at all.

When I had cried my heart out, as my aunt used to say, I stood up and turned away. I wiped my face with my white apron and blew my nose in the hankie from my pocket. I could see our breakfast was the worse for wear, and the boiled over coffee grounds were stuck to the stove lid.

I gathered my courage and looked at Jarvis. His tanned cheeks and the smile wrinkles at the edges of his eyes were wet.

"And what do you think of me now, Mr. Sim, after that fine performance?"

He took both my hands in his. "I'm thinking what I've always thought, for more than a year now. Just this Liz - I want to marry you."

MARRIED IN BLUE, YOU'LL ALWAYS BE TRUE

A few days later, I was the beautiful lady in blue, climbing into Jarvis Sim's truck on the farm and heading to the stone chapel we knew so well.

Linda had seen to it that a bouquet was waiting for me at the flower shop in the city, with a blue ribbon to match the dress. She insisted I needed "something old, something new, something borrowed, something blue". Before I moved to the farm, Jarvis picked up my sewing machine and a couple of boxes I had stored at Marj's. Included was the small package Ralph had delivered to me from Aunt Flo. It contained two wedding rings - her own, and one the army had returned to her. I asked Jarvis if he wanted to use them, and he was game. I washed the rings with Lux dish detergent and polished them with a soft cloth to renew the shine. So, Aunt Flo's wedding ring was my "something old". "Something new" was a lace hankie, just in case "Liz, the lady who never cries" needed it. "Something borrowed" was a pair of Linda's clip-on earrings that matched the rhinestones on the shoulder seams of my dress. And the "something blue" was, of course, my pretty wedding dress. Linda took a picture of us with her box camera just before we left the yard.

Jarvis had arranged everything with Rev. Bergen, the same minister who had conducted Wilma's funeral service. It was a warm day in July, the 18th, and the beautiful stone chapel was cool and exquisite. Perfect for a dream wedding.

Just before the ceremony, Marj drove up in her old car. She had promised to be my bridesmaid, and there she was, wearing a pretty blue dress and a wide smile. I had asked Jarvis if there was anyone he wanted to stand up with him. He grinned and said he would lean on old Rev. Bergen if he felt faint!

The wedding was over almost before it started. The "I do's", a scripture verse, a prayer, and the signing of our names. I would have liked music, but we did without it. We shook hands with Rev. Bergen and Marj hugged us both, promising to come and visit us in the Tansy Hills. Jarvis and I had an unspoken plan of where we were going. It was a sunny afternoon as we made our way to the cemetery, to Wilma's as yet unmarked grave. We took a moment, standing there together, silently thinking about her. She was the one who brought us together.

"My sister would approve," Jarvis said, his eyes smiling.

"Oh, she would for sure," I agreed, "She was hoping!"

I placed my bouquet at the head of the grave, and we left the quiet rows of crosses behind. As I looked back, the blue ribbon was moving in the breeze. Dear Wilma, still my friend. Death could never change that.

We went to a restaurant for supper, one that Jarvis had been to before, and the food was delicious. During our meal, he said it wasn't too late to change my mind about taking a trip to the Rocky Mountains.

When he had asked earlier, I said I preferred to stay at home, and maybe we could look at it for next year as a first-anniversary celebration. Banff was a popular honeymoon destination. I remembered some visitors to the hospital last year who had just come from there. The woman was wearing sunglasses, a wide-brimmed hat, and white pedal pushers, with a striped t-shirt. They gave the impression of being rich and stuck-up. I could imagine Jarvis and me touring around Banff among people like that, and I just didn't want to risk the awkward feeling. We were no better and no worse than anyone else. I believed that, but I sometimes wondered when people looked at me, if they suspected I was from the hospital. Maybe my reluctance to go was simply that I wanted to spend this first summer on the farm. Besides, there was someone on my mind, someone who might need us in the next couple of weeks.

I told Jarvis how much I liked his truck. He said, "Well it's *our* truck now and tomorrow, I'm going to teach you to drive."

I burst out laughing, too loud, too long. "Oh golly, you're a brave husband! There is something else I'm hoping to learn. Wilma said you have her accordion. Someday, when you are way in the back forty, I'm going to see if I can squeeze some music out of that thing."

"Okay, and if you do, I'll dust off my fiddle and we can form a family band!"

We drove into the lane, and the place looked different. I was trying to spot the change, when I realized the transformation wasn't in the farmyard. Of course, it wasn't. It was somewhere within me, and my sense of belonging.

Jarvis nailed it as he parked beside the house. "So now you really are a farmer's wife. Welcome home."

Linda appeared on the step, and called to us with a wide smile. "Good evening, Mr. and Mrs. Sim! Step inside, your wedding cake awaits you!"

The girl had outdone herself. Candles and wild roses adorned the kitchen table along with a decorated cake. As she turned to rush out the door, I grabbed her by the shoulders and pulled her in for a hug.

"Thank you, Linda. You're such a romantic."

"As are you, Liz Sim!"

Linda had already taken care of the few evening chores. Jarvis and I strolled down the lane and around the yard, holding hands, each with our own thoughts. I remembered that I once wrote a note to a little girl when both our lives were falling apart. It was back in January '56 when I left my job at Cleavers in disgrace. Only five words on the note: "Hold on to your dreams." They were written for both of us, with a very faint hope on a very dark day. Somehow, I had held on since that day, not even sure what I was holding on to, but it had been worth it. My dreams had come true. Despite disappointment and tragedy, that dim hope had flickered, survived, and burst into flame on my wedding day.

I turned to Jarvis and asked, "Do you want to know why I wanted to be married on this date?"

"Tell me."

I kissed him on the cheek. "Because today is my 34th birthday, and I get to begin a new year with my brand-new husband!"

TILL DEATH DO US PART

The next morning, Jarvis said we needed to go back into Stillwater to buy a birthday gift for me. I told him I already owned the whole world, and there wasn't a thing I could dream of or wish for. But my husband was a determined man, and had a plan. Off we went, arriving in the city well before noon. Jarvis was a man on a mission.

We entered a jewelry store, he made his purchase, and we were out of there in less than fifteen minutes. So sweetly circling my neck was an exquisite string of pearls. Jarvis wouldn't let me watch when he paid for them, and I shuddered to think of the cost. The jeweler assured us they were real, each pearl formed so miraculously by nature. Although the pearls were matched in size for the necklace, we could see each was a beautiful creation in itself, slightly different from the one beside it.

I had never owned anything truly beautiful. Just before we left the store, the elderly jeweler who completed the sale smiled at me and said, "Don't store them away, my dear. Pearls love to be worn." I could see myself wearing them every day while gathering eggs, baking bread, and working in the garden. I might even "wear them out" from overuse.

Jarvis was pleased with his purchase. "Pearls stand for wisdom, Liz. Did you know that?"

For a girl who had spent eight years in the hospital for the mentally ill, this was the ultimate compliment. I did not think of myself as wise, but I was wise enough to be grateful.

We passed a bakery two doors down from the jewelers, and stopped to watch as a machine dropped donuts into hot oil to cook them. We bought a half dozen, piping hot, and headed to the truck.

Jarvis started the motor. "Today is your birthday celebration. Where do you want to go for lunch?"

I didn't have to think twice. "Buck's Diner, if you please."

The pie maker himself noticed us drive into the parking lot, and rushed out the door to meet us.

"It's you, Goh-jus! And the word on the street is that my best girl just got married!"

I couldn't help grinning from ear to ear, "You bet I did!"

Buck pushed my chair in for me as I sat down, and he commented, "Beautiful pearls - for a beautiful lady."

My cup was full. I was in love with my life, with being a wife, and in love with Jarvis Sim for the rest of my days. Buck had added a jukebox to the diner. Perfect! He went to the machine, dropped in a quarter and soon the strains of "Moonlight Becomes You" filled the room. I recognized that one - Bing Crosby, 1942. Romantic old Buck had chosen that song to celebrate our news. I hummed along as we waited for our lunch.

I looked across the table at my handsome husband, and I was reminded of Shakespeare's words, "The world is my oyster." Those words summed up that moment for me. Maybe the oyster quote came to my mind because of the lovely pearls around my neck.

I leaned towards Jarvis, and whispered, "There's nothing more I could wish for. I have it all!"

We ate the donuts on the way home, and as we neared the town of Tansy, Jarvis commented, "Well, it won't be long now."

"What won't?"

"Your first truck driving lesson!"

Oh, help! I had forgotten about his threat to teach me to drive. Why ruin a perfect special day!

Seeing the look on my face, he squelched any excuses I was fumbling for. "Today's the day. And you're gonna love it."

We turned off the road and into our yard. Each time I viewed our yard from the lane, I had a happy feeling all over again. I had longed to live on a farm, and our cozy farmhouse was my dream come true.

Buddy lazily got up to greet us from his shady spot on the north side of the house. Jarvis was coming around to the passenger side. I took my cue and shakily got out. Slowly, I walked around the front of the truck, stopped to rub Buddy's head, and finally hoisted myself up behind the steering wheel.

I tried to think logically. How hard could it be? It probably wasn't that much different than running a sewing machine! My husband was talking, and I welcomed the instructions - starter, clutch, gearshift, gas pedal, brake.

Jarvis was so happy to be sharing his truck, and I didn't want to let him down. I listened to every word he said, but I didn't hear a thing!

He sat in the middle of the bench seat, close enough, I hoped, to rescue us if I ran amok. He appeared to be very relaxed.

"Okay, start 'er up." Just to complicate it, there was a foot pedal starter, but all right, I got the motor humming. Jarvis said he figured I would be more at ease driving in the pasture, rather than on the road. Truer words were never spoken! He explained what I had to do - put my foot on the clutch, run the gear shift, ease off the clutch, and give it a little gas.

I was breathing deep. We shot forward and jerked to halt. Okay, cancel that. Try again, getting the idea. The next time, we inched forward a little, and before I could kill the engine again, Jarvis said, "Give 'er some gas."

That's when all heck broke loose! I tramped it, and that yellow streak rocketed forward straight for the pasture. My hands froze to the wheel, my foot to the gas pedal. There was no help for it. We were going into orbit any minute. I didn't dare look across at Jarvis, so I will never know what he was thinking or doing.

We hit the closed barbed wire gate full force, and I heard a zing as the wire whistled past my side window. Oh, my land, this was a runaway train wreck, and there was no stop button! I thought if I turned the steering wheel just a touch, we might slow down. Well, we didn't, but we veered off the pasture road, and headed straight for the slough. I squeezed my eyes shut and heard the willows bunching up under the truck. In two minutes, I had wedged that beautiful baby into so much muck and debris that we came to a lurching stop. I put my head on the steering wheel. I heard Jarvis slide out of the passenger door.

What a short marriage! Two days. Over almost before it started. Well, I wouldn't trade these two days of being Mrs. Jarvis Sim for every pearl in the land.

I lifted my forehead off the steering wheel and caught a glimpse of Jarvis bent over at the back of his beloved and precious truck. Probably surveying the damages… or could he be conducting its funeral? I could see he was shaking - with rage likely, or maybe he was sobbing.

Never one to avoid facing up to my sins, I bailed out and stepped precariously on bent-over willow trees, aiming to get to the back of the truck.

I couldn't wait to apologize, so I yelled from where I was, "Jarvis, I'm so sorry! I'll be sorry till the day I die! I'll buy you a new truck, if I have to work till I'm 100."

I noticed he was standing now, and I was getting closer. I'd be heading back to the hospital, there was no question about that. I'd sleep there tonight, back where I belonged. I had landed there twice already. Three times is a charm.

Tears were running down his face. I was still yelling, even though I was standing in front of him by that time. I hollered, "Are you hurt? Are you hurt bad?"

He burst out laughing.

"Lizzie, that was quite a ride!"

Was he laughing? I couldn't tell. He grabbed my hand and started marching us back to the house.

"Are you taking me back to the hospital now?"

"The hospital? No, of course not! We're going for the tractor to pull the truck out of the slough."

"Is it wrecked?"

"Nope, just got the carbon cleared out of the pipes and maybe a little scratch or two on the paint."

I was stuck on how mad he must be. "Do you want a divorce?"

"Never, Lizzie, never!"

I had been called Liz all my life, sometimes "Lizard" back in my school days, and Elizabeth Rose the day I was born, but not Lizzie.

He finally saw then that I was seriously upset, so he stopped and put his hands on my shoulders. He looked me in the eyes. "My only regret is that I didn't meet you sooner, Lizzie. My life has been far too dull without you!"

Later in the day, I wondered what to make for supper. We'd had a filling lunch at Buck's Diner and munched on donuts on the way home. That was enough for me. I asked Jarvis if he was hungry, and he said, "Oh, let's just have toast and a cup of coffee. I think I'm livin' on love!"

THE SHIVAREE

I thought I saw the flash of headlights across the bedroom ceiling, then nothing. It was Saturday night, two days after our wedding, and I had almost fallen asleep when I heard a whisper, "Get up you guys - it's a shivaree!"

No mistake. The racket had wakened Jarvis, and we could hear men and women chanting, "Shivaree, shivaree, shivaree!" They circled our house, banging on pots and pans and ringing a cowbell.

The whispered warning came from Linda at the screened window. "Alfred Miller is here. You know what he's like. He'll go in the house and climb in bed with you, so you'd better come out!"

Jarvis was annoyed and grumbling to himself as he pulled on his pants and buttoned his shirt. I grabbed his denim jacket from the hook by the door, and fastened it over my nightgown. I shoved my feet into my shoes on the way outside. We stood together on our step as the last of the parade came around the corner of the house. Our brave guard dog, Buddy, was chasing the merrymakers, barking, and enjoying the excitement.

We peered into the darkness and tried to make out the scene. Linda slipped into the house behind us and turned on the yard light. As the area lit up, we saw a swarm of Jarvis' friends and neighbors who had come to celebrate our marriage. Jarvis looked different without his glasses, but Linda was on the ball and fetched them.

Alfred was the loudest of everyone. I found out he was a friend from the old playing-for-dances days when Jarvis was young. His banjo was strung around his neck. Another man, Jim Bender, had a guitar. They struck up the band. A long table was unloaded from the back of a truck and set up near the house. It was quickly laden with food and gifts. Some people sat on the tailgate of a truck, some on a bench, already making themselves at home.

I wondered what these neighbors were thinking of me, and then I realized it wasn't about *me*. It was about *us*! I was introduced to some of the ladies who told me they figured a surprise party would be best so Jarvis couldn't wiggle out of it. Celebrating with a noisy, old-fashioned shivaree was pretty much a thing of the past, but friends and neighbors decided to go with the idea, just for the fun of it.

Linda soon interrupted our conversation and pulled me back to where Jarvis was. Some couples were dancing. There was no moon, but the stars were out. Alfred and Jim played one of my favorites, "For Me and My Gal". Music trivia went off in my head - Judy Garland and Gene Kelly, 1942.

A warm sense of community settled over me as Jim Bender led the group in the familiar song, "Side by Side". The song brought back memories of my friends and neighbors the town of Cala when I was young. I was eager to get to know these new friends here in the Tansy Hills. The singing continued with peppy songs like "Roll out the Barrel", and just to be Alfred, he finished off with his rendition of "All Shook Up", a brand-new release by Elvis Presley.

Lunch was served, and it was a grand layout - jelly roll, matrimony cake, oatmeal cookies, and butter tarts. Coffee and cups magically appeared, and the fun lasted about an hour. I could see a long line of cars lined up on the side of the lane, and extending down the road. They had driven in with their lights off to surprise us.

When the music stopped, Alfred yelled, "Speech! Speech!" For once, it wasn't my place to do the talking. Jarvis stepped up and held our joined hands high in the air between us. "I'm the luckiest guy in the world! Thanks for coming!"

Short and sweet. There was loud applause and whistling (probably by Alfred) and then it was over. The best night of my life? I think it was.

We walked with our visitors as they returned to their vehicles. Alfred headed down the road in the dark, playing the banjo all the way to his truck. There were invitations galore to come and visit. Marie Bender introduced herself and walked with me down the lane.

She said, "I'm really looking forward to getting to know you, Liz. All of us are so happy for both of you."

The celebration was true Saskatchewan hospitality at its finest. We stood in the yard, while each one backed out and turned around, and we were still waving as the last tail light disappeared. The party was officially over. We had been shivareed!

As we turned toward the house, I said to Jarvis, "I never dreamed I would meet all the neighbors while wearing my nightgown!"

"They didn't give us much choice on that, did they?" Suddenly, to my surprise, I was scooped up in the air and carried over the threshold into the kitchen.

IT'S NOT THE END

During the next couple of weeks, I figured out that Linda was pregnant, as I had suspected. She had completely stopped her incessant talk about Bob and the fun they were having in the summer holidays. She had not told her parents. Old familiar feelings flooded my mind. Dear Linda, I'm so sorry.

"Does Bob know?"

"He does. I told him on Wednesday. He turned sulky, and said we probably should break up then. He wouldn't talk about it, wouldn't discuss what we should do. He tore out of the yard, tires squealing, dust flying. I guess it's my problem. Saturday night I saw him driving around town with Mary, the one we call 'everybody's friend'."

I put my arm around her. She was so young and defenseless. This was adult stuff, and she was just a kid.

"I had such big plans, Liz. I thought Bob and I would have a long engagement. I'd go to Normal School and I'd be a teacher after we were married. Now all I'll be is the biggest fool in the country."

Linda cried a lot. I promised I would be with her every step of the way. I told her it feels like the end of the world, but it isn't. I know, because I've been there.

She was shocked. "You, Liz? You had a baby?"

"I did. It doesn't need to destroy you. You're just as good as the next one. Don't forget that!" I hugged her. "We're going through this one together."

When I told Jarvis, he didn't seem surprised. "There's an unanswered question I've had for years. The gossips always have a lot to say about unwed mothers. Why do they have nothing to say about unmarried fathers?" I'd had the same question.

The following Sunday morning, Linda arrived on our doorstep with red-rimmed eyes. As soon as she saw me, she burst out crying, shaking with deep sobs as I hugged her.

"Dad kicked me out." His last words to me were, "Don't bother coming back."

"And your mom?"

"She's mad. She's mad at Dad and at me and at Bob. Mad about what the neighbors will say."

"She might come around. Anger comes first. For most people, it's easier to get mad than to cry."

"Oh, she sure wasn't crying. I was the only one doing that!"

When Jarvis came in the door, Linda quickly put her arms on the table and rested her head there to hide her tears. He raised his eyebrows in a silent question to me, asking, "Have you invited her to stay?"

I shook my head and pointed to him. His voice was husky as he touched the girl's shoulder.

"Linda, you better go take a look at the guest house. Liz has it all ready for you."

EPILOGUE

(For Eden)

I drove the truck into Cleaver's lane on a Sunday afternoon in lilac time. Their neat and orderly yard was lined with blossoming shrubs, and a large garden already showed rows and rows of vegetables. Jarvis and I thought of phoning ahead, but I wanted the option to chicken out at the gate if I couldn't follow through. It had been three years since I was transported away from this place to the Psych Ward, and I wondered almost every day since then what the Cleaver family thought of me. I had seen Dot briefly at the hospital when she came to visit and she forgave me. I hoped the rest would, too.

It was Robert who approached us as we were getting out of the vehicle. He looked quizzically at Jarvis, and then at me.

"Liz! Liz Parker!" He exclaimed, reaching his right hand towards me.

"Yes, it's me, Robert, but I'm Liz Sim now. Meet Jarvis, my better half."

Farmers are never stuck for words. The weather, the crops, it doesn't matter, being friendly is their second nature. When I heard Jarvis ask, "You getting much rain up here?" I knew I was free to go find the kids. I didn't have to search. They were coming out of various corners of the yard, curious as to who would be visiting on a Sunday afternoon, driving a yellow truck.

Roy was first. He was vigorously rubbing his hands with an oily rag, as he met me near his car. I had noticed an old banged-up car when we drove in, front doors wide open and the radio cranked up. The hood was raised, and I guessed Roy was tinkering with the engine, just as I would have expected him to. That lopsided grin grabbed my heart.

"You grew up, Roy!"

He sighed and half frowned. "I'm workin' on it."

"That your car?"

"It's my dream! And I see you're driving, too!"

I have always told on myself. I can't help it. Pointing to Jarvis, I said, "I nearly killed that good man the first time I got behind the wheel." Roy laughed, and thought I was kidding, but it was closer to the truth than he knew.

Dot tore out of the kitchen door and raced towards me. What the heck! I ran too, and we met in the middle. I hugged that girl like there was no tomorrow.

"Liz, it's you! I can't believe you came!"

One by one, the rest of the family joined us in their rustic summer kitchen. The cookstove had seen better days, but a rhubarb cake had just come out of the oven, and we could smell coffee bubbling. Our arrival was good timing.

Will quickly sat on the bench beside me. He was warm and friendly, and he was a looker all right!

I tried to remember how old he would be. "Are you in high school?"

"Grade 10. I'm 16. We all go to school in town now on the bus. They closed Briar Rose, so Mac will never get a chance to ride to school by horse and buggy."

Speaking of Mac, there he was, boldly standing in front of me. He had an announcement to make. "Roy bought me and Nick a horse!"

"He did! Well, blow me down! What a great brother you've got!"

Nick piped up, eyes shining with pride, "He bought it out of his first paycheck from the garage."

"Well, let's go see this mighty horse!"

They ran ahead of me to the corral beside the barn and whistled. There he was, trotting towards us. A perfect pony, just the right size. He was brown with a white star, and a very long mane and tail.

"Oh, he's a beauty! What's his name?"

Nicky glanced at my face, and with almost a smirk he answered, "Buckshot!" We burst out laughing. It was wild Bill Hickok's steed. We both remembered that!

After we had been there for a while, I noticed a little girl on the sidelines, handling a little kitten, none too gently. She and Dot rather suddenly disappeared into the house, and when they emerged, the girl's face had been washed and her red hair brushed and tied in a ponytail. The kitten was gone. Likely it had escaped under a bed.

Dot presented her sister. "This is Rosie." Of course. Maggie was expecting when she and Dot came to the hospital to visit me.

"Hi Rosie. I bet you are the darling of the family!"

She glanced at various family members, as if hoping someone would agree with me. No one paid any attention until Rosie's dad pulled her up on his knee, and with a smile, handed her his spoon. She looked around the table with a grin, and dug into his rhubarb cake. That little interaction was perhaps the best for me of the whole day. I had hoped that man would find happiness again, and share it with his wonderful pack of kids.

Dot wanted to talk, to tell me everything, just as she had on the day we met on ward 3C. "Did you know I named Rosie? I named her after you."

I didn't think she was serious. "You did?"

"I did. Maggie said if it was a girl, I could make the choice. So I called her Elizabeth Rose."

My heart stopped. Sometimes when something so sweet and so good covers something so hard and so painful, there is a healing that takes place, completely and forever. I remembered the big new patch I sewed over the ripped one on John McDonalds's overalls. The old tatter was never to be seen again. I would never again resent the name Irene had chosen for Marie. Little Elizabeth Rose had been named for me, with love from Dot. And what an interesting little namesake! Rosie was downing rhubarb cake, her orange freckles sprinkled all over her pale face. I could already see a pretty little dress taking shape at my sewing machine somewhere around Christmas time.

Maggie said very little, but she smiled a time or two, and I could see she was more confident than when I met her before. She made a second pot of coffee when we drained the first one. I complimented her on the yard and garden, and she admitted she would rather work outside than in. There was something about her that puzzled me, something I couldn't pinpoint. My aunt used to say, "There's more here than meets the eye."

Another surprise was coming. Mac told me, loud enough for the rest to hear, "I can still sing."

I figured someone had put him up to this, as I doubted he remembered singing with me. He was only three years old when I left.

I didn't want to put him on the spot, so I said, "I know a song we need to sing for Maggie."

It was one we used to sing - "If I Knew You Were Comin', I'd Have Baked a Cake".

Mac didn't miss a beat, he joined right in. Word for word, line for line, he remembered!

Mac and I clapped for our performance, as did the rest. I suggested Nick go find a syrup pail of cookies in the truck. For old times' sake, I'd baked raisin cookies. That was the kind I'd made on my first day as their housekeeper. Nick passed them around, even though we'd just eaten cake, as there is no end to a farm family's appetite.

Before we left, Dot put what was left of the cookies into the cake pan. She asked me to walk down the lane, where she gathered lilac blooms for me, and filled the red and white syrup pail with them. I once said to her, "I'll tell you what Dot, never return a pan without putting something in it. That shows you're a good neighbor." She had remembered.

In true Saskatchewan style, the whole family walked to the truck with us. Jarvis reached for my hand as we walked. I still wondered what Robert was thinking. The last time he saw me, I was in bad shape. Did he think I was still crazy? Maybe Jarvis felt my discomfort. When Will asked how long we had been married, Jarvis had a fine answer.

"Almost two years. Best day of my life when I met this girl."

Dot pressed her arm against me, and turned her eyes to the sky. She had already told me she thought he was handsome.

Jarvis drove slowly down the lane, and I waved until we turned on to the main road. My cup was full to the brim, and I had a song in my heart.

The Cleaver family had not only survived, they had thrived. And so had I.

ACKNOWLEDGEMENTS

Thank you to my readers! I appreciate your feedback and suggestions. Please keep in touch at **dotontheprairie@gmail.com**

Thank you to my Team: siblings, extended family, and so many friends for cheering me on!

Thank you Sunny, for unfailing love and digital expertise.

Thank you Daylin, for your videography and technical support.

Thank you, Lantern Hill Communications, for editing and proofreading.

Thank you, my brother Jon, for your gift of the song, "Sure as the River". So true! The answer is love.

SONG: SURE AS THE RIVER

Jon Sloan 2021©

Just as sure as the sun shines down on us all
As sure as the stars shine above
And as sure as the river rolls down to the sea
You will find the answer is love

Days can be filled with doubts and with fears
And you wonder which way to go
Nights can be lonely when you're all by yourself
And you wonder, does anyone know?

Just as sure as the sun shines down on us all
And as sure as the stars shine above
And as sure as the river rolls down to the sea
You will find the answer is love

Love will carry you through the years
No matter where you may roam
And as sure as the river rolls down to sea
Love will carry you home

Just as sure as the sun shines down on us all
And as sure as the stars shine above
And as sure as the river rolls down to the sea
You will find the answer is love
I John 4:16

SONGS IN THE
PUBLIC DOMAIN

Billy Boy, 1824, Traditional Nursery Rhyme
Jesus Loves Me, 1859, Anna Bartlett Warner
Leaning on the Everlasting Arms, 1887, Elisha A. Hoffman
Little Brown Jug, 1869, Traditional
Old Lady Leary, 1871, Traditional Nursery Rhyme
Put on your Old Gray Bonnet, 1909, Percy Wenrich
Shelter in the Time of Storm, 1885, Ira D. Sankey
Twilight is Falling, 1881, Aldine S. Kieffer

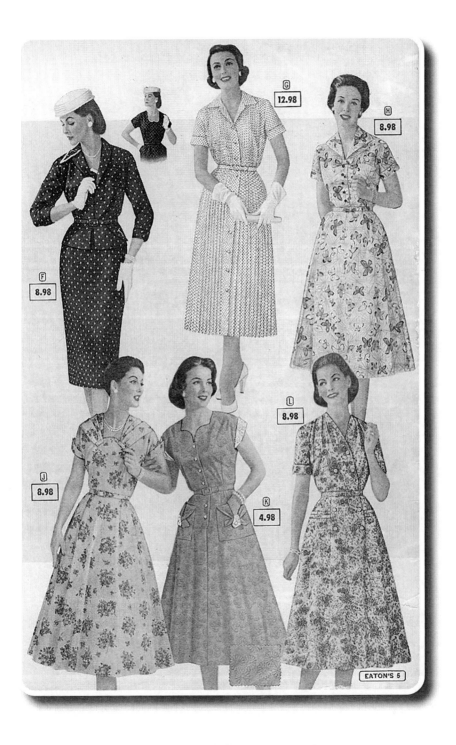

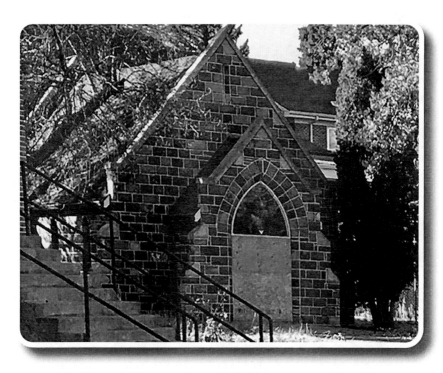

Photo by Trudy Ramsay

Just around the corner...
Guess what! There's a brand-new book on the way! It is the third in the series, *Wandering Back to Saskatchewan*.

We met Maggie in the first two books, **Dot on the Prairie** and **Sure as the River**. What do you think of her?
Maggie may well have been your least favorite person. People are the way they are for so many reasons...
Coming soon, Maggie's story:

Something to Say

Wandering Back to Saskatchewan
By Charlotte Evelyn Sloan
Dot on the Prairie
Sure as the River
Something to Say